Reign

A Guide to Ruling Your Inner Kingdom of Self
with Grace, Power, and Authenticity

MARY KRYGIEL

Illustrations by Jen Yoon | www.jenyoonart.com

Publishing services provided by 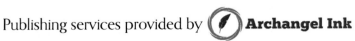 Archangel Ink

ISBN: 978-1-950043-19-4

Acknowledgments

A very special thanks to the helpers who have been with me on this journey. This book would not have come together without your support. Thank you for offering your encouragement, insight, and guidance at exactly the right time.

Ella Krygiel, Laura Packer, Jen Yoon, Elissa Savos, Sammy Savos, the amazing team at Archangel Ink, and my wonderful husband, Rich Krygiel.

For my husband, Rich, and my children, Zack and Ella.

Contents

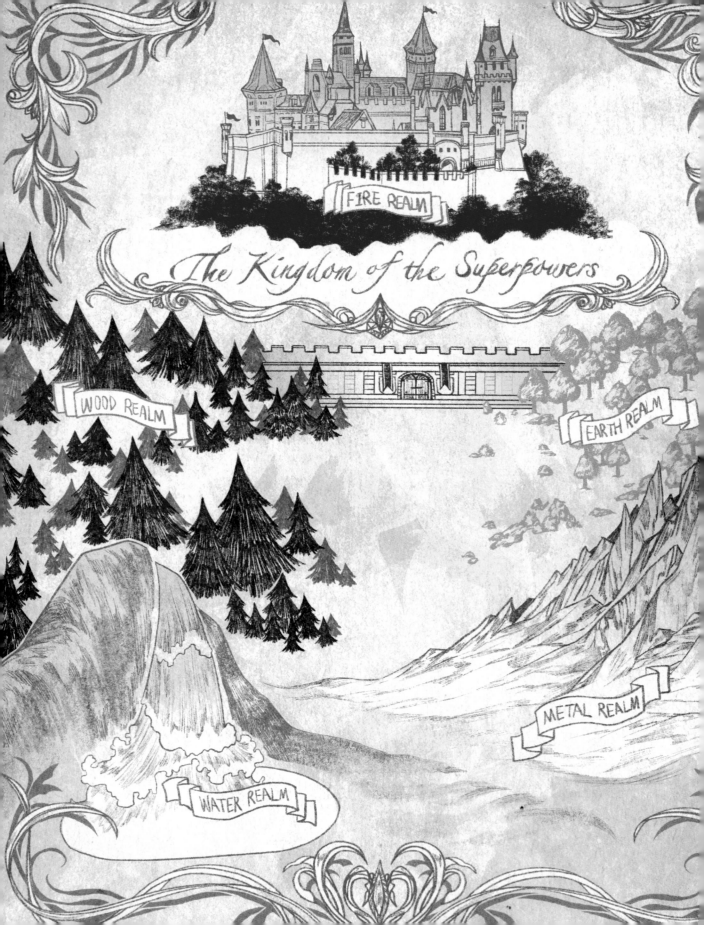

Introduction

Life is a series of natural and spontaneous changes. Don't resist them—that only creates sorrow.

–Lao Tzu

The ancient Chinese observed nature over centuries and discovered an inherent life force that powers all of life's processes, called qi (pronounced "chee"). This force is best seen in the changing seasons. Earth's landscape transforms from one season to the next in a process that continues unhindered year after year. After witnessing these seasonal changes over time, the ancient Chinese understood that humans should work with the flow of nature's transformations rather than against it.

Living close to the land, they knew there was an appropriate time in each season to take action. Life was easier for them when they followed this flow of movement. Often, their lives depended upon it. For example, not harvesting crops before a devastating frost could lead to a long, hungry winter. By living in harmony with this flow of nature, they understood each season had a purpose: spring was a time to plan and plant the season's crops; summer was a time to gather outside to work with others and exchange information; late summer was a time to reap the harvest and share bounty and burdens; autumn was a time to prepare the ground for the next season and acknowledge what went well in the previous one; and winter was a time to rest and reflect before the next cycle began. Adapting and working with each seasonal change was like floating downstream with the current of life force.

They applied this same philosophy of following the natural flow of life to their interactions with others. Just as they worked with the seasons in their farming livelihood, they recognized that there is an *appropriate time* to speak, act, or be silent in every relationship. By following the same rhythm of the seasonal changes when interacting with others, they found their relationships were more rewarding. They understood that there is a time to plan and create change (like spring); a time to laugh and engage (like summer); a time to nurture, share, and enjoy life's goodness (like the harvest time); a time to acknowledge what is good and let go of what is not (like autumn); and a time to simply be quiet and thoughtful (like winter).

In our modern-day context, we could certainly learn from this perspective. Rather than follow the

1

natural cycle of the ancient Chinese, we often sabotage it. Specifically, social media has provided an almost incessant call to answer the rapid sharing of images and information. As much as this sharing allows for community and connectedness, the desire to participate in it can also lead to a self-presentation that may not always be grounded in authenticity.

Moving through such a shift in authenticity pits us against the flow of nature's life force. It's like a favorite pair of jeans that fit perfectly when first purchased but become too snug or stylistically outdated with the passing of time: this overuse or underuse of a person's constitutional energy can start to feel uncomfortable. When you look in the mirror at the too-tight jeans, you have a choice to make: continue to wear ill-fitting clothing or search the closet for a more appropriate alternative. If your usual or forced attitude, comments, and way of being are becoming like the outdated or snug pair of jeans, this can be a call to change.

The purpose of the journey through the Kingdom of the Superpowers is to explore this possibility of change. As the ancient Chinese found, *nature is change*. Once movement stops, stagnation occurs and, eventually, decay begins. Shifts in authenticity are roadblocks that slow or prevent the natural forward progression of one's life path. On this journey through the Kingdom of the Superpowers, consider if there are any obstacles present on your own path that might be preventing you from moving forward to be your best, most authentic self.

A Guidebook for the Journey to the Kingdom of the Superpowers

Before any journey is begun, it's best to spend time preparing. Whether this takes the form of updating a passport, learning about local customs, or just checking the weather, a little bit of planning and forethought can go a long way toward making the trip a more pleasant one. This guidebook will offer helpful tips and practical advice for your journey to the Kingdom of the Superpowers.

History of the Land and the Five Elements

The Kingdom of the Superpowers is steeped in the rich history of the Chinese. Over many centuries, the ancient Chinese observed and studied nature. As farmers, they lived close to the land and watched for subtle changes in weather patterns. They found that there are five changing seasons on earth. In addition to what we know today as the four seasons, the ancient Chinese witnessed a fifth season between summer and autumn called the harvest season. This harvest season is a time that begins in mid-August and ends in late October. Since crops were harvested during this time, the ancient Chinese saw this period as its own distinct season.

Within each of the five seasons, the ancient Chinese saw energetic movement. They paired these five directional movements to five everyday elements: wood, fire, earth, metal, and water. Each season was named for what they determined to be its corresponding energetic movement: spring = wood, summer = fire, harvest season = earth, autumn = metal, winter = water. The ancient Chinese observed that the movements occurring within each season are like certain processes in the body: a child's upward growth is like a tree growing in springtime, and sleeping is like a dormant seed in winter.

This pairing of the seasons with the five elements eventually developed over time into what is now referred to as the Law of the Five Elements. The Law of the Five Elements became a basis for understanding all of life's processes, including human functioning, and is one of the principles of modern-day acupuncture. The Kingdom of the Superpowers comprises five realms, each named for one of these five elements.

Understanding the Kingdom Infrastructure

The earliest written textbook of acupuncture is from 100 BCE. In that ancient time, China was composed of kingdoms, and every individual would serve a specific role in support of their kingdom (the nobility, the generals, the treasurers, the gardeners, etc.). Each person would do their job. All roles were needed in order to keep the kingdom flourishing, and there would be little transfer of responsibilities between roles. The gardener wouldn't be asked to be an advisor to a noble, for example, nor would the treasurer serve as a gatekeeper.

By studying the five elements so closely, the ancient Chinese detected twelve specific functions within those five elements that serve to help keep nature in balance. The kingdom infrastructure was their framework for understanding these twelve functions of life that are observed in nature. These twelve natural functions serve distinct and unique purposes in order to keep nature on a pattern of continued, healthy growth and progress.

Because this kingdom infrastructure was how they saw life, they applied it to their understanding of the functioning of humans. Each person is their own separate kingdom. Therefore, within every individual there are twelve specific energetic movements functioning simultaneously in support of the body. If a person is experiencing physical pain or emotional distress, at least one of the twelve energetic movements is blocked. Put another way, if there is chronic stress or anxiety, one or more of the twelve energetic workers are not doing their job properly in the person's individual kingdom. The Kingdom of the Superpowers has five realms named for each element, and each realm is home to some of the twelve superpowers.

Cultural Expectations and Rules of Engagement

There are universal cultural and social norms in the Kingdom of the Superpowers. Using a superpower is a gift of influence in society and must be respected. Over time, the following rules and expectations were developed for the proper use of all twelve superpowers.

1. Our greatest strength is also our greatest weakness.

Despite there being twelve superpowers available to support a person in every moment, there is only *one* of these twelve powers—a home base—that each person will naturally gravitate toward using more than the other eleven. A key tenet of the Law of the Five Elements is the idea that everyone is born with a primary temperament, or way of being. Having strength in one of the twelve superpowers over the other eleven indicates one's primary temperament. The use of this one superpower gives a person their greatest strength and power in life. However, with overuse or underuse, it can also become their greatest weakness.

The question is, how does one know where their greatest power lies? If you observe your ways of being, language, and attitude over time, it becomes apparent that *one* of the twelve energies feels like a home base to you. It may be that several of them call to you, but there will likely be one energetic super suit that you choose to wear time and time again as a practiced habit.

2. With great power comes great responsibility.

One might argue that to wear a different energetic way of being, or energetic super suit, is to be phony or inauthentic. However, it is quite the opposite. To curb or deny your natural powers is a false manner of being and will cause pain and discomfort on many levels over time. It takes courage to change even the smallest thing. The mind can quickly talk you out of actions that may make you feel the slightest bit uncomfortable. Utilizing one of your twelve superpowers may feel uncomfortable at first but will eventually become second nature with continued use and practice.

We've all learned about cultural and social norms over time. For example, funerals are a solemn, respectful time of grief, parties and celebrations are boisterous and joyful, and libraries are quiet and contemplative. In each of these venues or events, we adjust our behavior to an appropriate level based on outward circumstances and learned expectations.

In everyday life, moments pass rapidly, and each moment is an occasion to adjust our energetic way of being in order to provide ease with ourselves and those around us. We can do this by changing our one worn-out way of being and wearing one of our other eleven super suits. All twelve are always at our disposal.

3. Seek to weaken aggressive powers.

Each of the twelve superpowers serves a purpose in the kingdom. No single superpower is more important than another. Unfortunately, that doesn't stop a superpower from becoming greedy and trying to dominate the others by using its power at inopportune times. Like choosing to dress inappropriately for a formal event, it's wearing the wrong super suit on an important mission.

The good news is that nature has put in place an instinctive check to balance these overbearing tendencies. When one superpower tries to dominate, nature creates a reaction from a controlling element in order to limit that effort. This can be seen in nature's five elements: water can put out fire, metal can cut through overgrown forests, earth can be used to channel or dam water, fire can melt metal, and wood's roots can hold earth in place. These contrary powers are like a natural kryptonite to limit power excess. This natural controlling cycle tries to ensure that all twelve superpowers are used without prejudice within each person's individual kingdom.

4. Seek to amplify weak powers.

Just as nature has implemented a plan to control excess aggressive energy, it has simultaneously allowed for a strengthening function for weaker powers. Each element has a mother realm that encourages and empowers its child. This phenomenon is a basic principle of the Law of the Five Elements. Like a child that needs a mother's comfort after a fall or small injury, a weak element can seek strength from its mother in times of need. The ancient Chinese observed this in their daily life: wood can start a fire, fire's ashes enrich the earth, the earth houses and maintains precious metals, metals enrich the quality of water, and water is needed for plants and trees (the source of wood) to grow. By strengthening what is weak, the empowering ability works to sustain the health of a person's kingdom.

Tools for the Journey to the Kingdom of the Superpowers

In addition to reading the guidebook, it's important to pack a few essential tools in order to make the journey to the land of the superpowers a successful one.

Map

The illustrated map outlines the kingdom and the direction to each superpower home.

Scroll of Meditations

The Scroll of Meditations provides an inspirational meditation for each of the twelve superpowers. Meditating on a superpower before actually encountering it provides an appreciation of the spirit of its energy.

Lexicon of Powers

The Lexicon of Powers is a simple chart of all of the superpowers and their strengths and weaknesses. It should be consulted before venturing into a superpower territory.

Lastly, the most important tool to bring with you on this journey is the intention for personal introspection. As you travel through the kingdom, pay attention to places where you feel more or less comfortable. Some areas will be familiar to you while others will feel like a strange land. Embark with an open mind. At the end of each chapter, there are tools for strengthening and developing your superpowers. Each one of you will have your own interpretation in how to best channel your twelve gifts. There is no right way! Use this guidebook and the prompts as a starting place for meditation, journaling, or self-reflection.

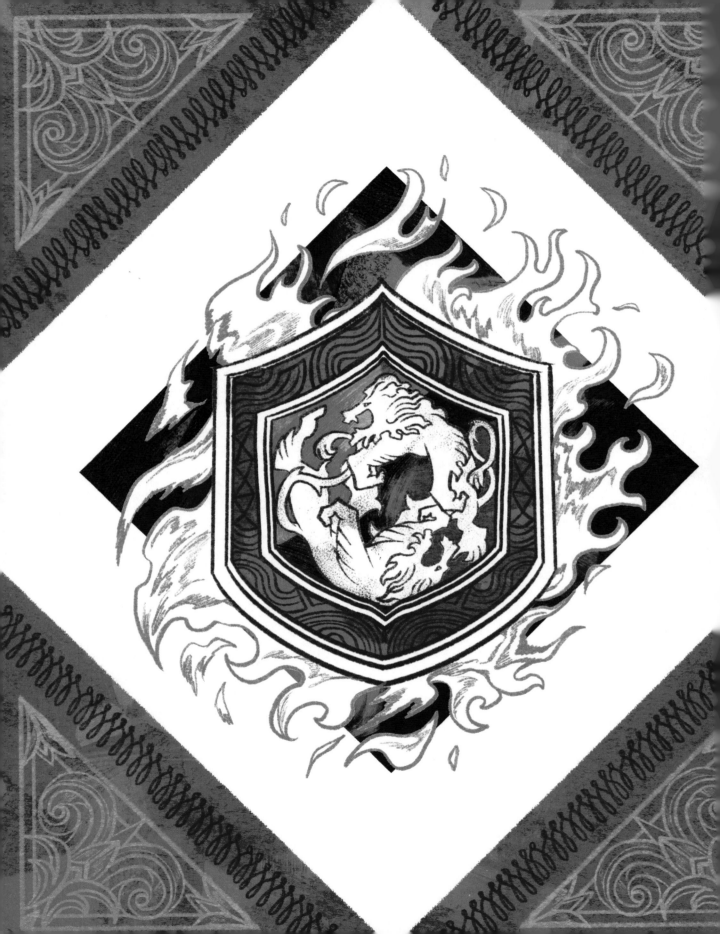

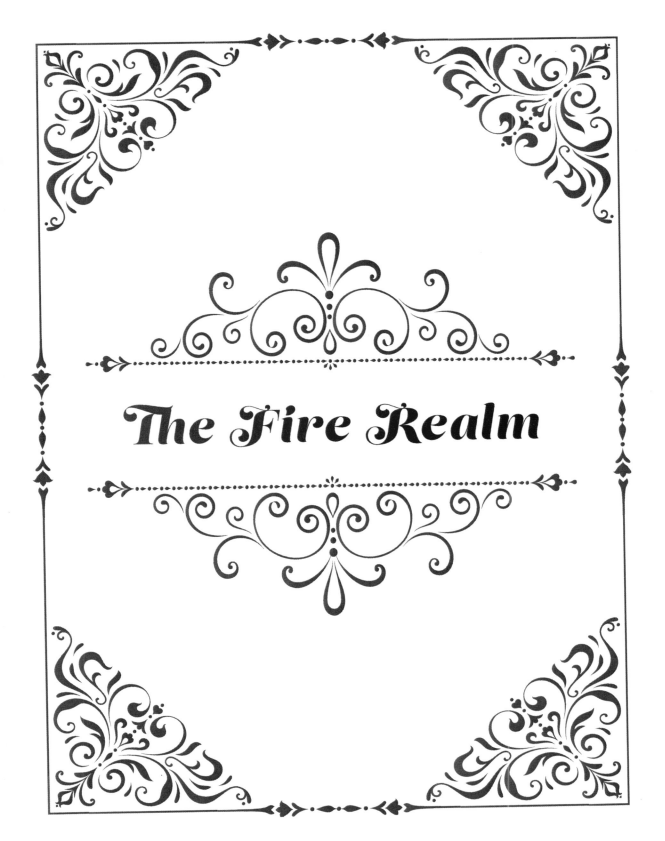

The Fire Realm

Gifts of the Realm

Social Connection – Vulnerability – Discernment – Love

The journey begins at the Fire Realm, which is vast and holds four out of the twelve superpowers. Not only is the Fire Realm the largest of all of the realms, but it's also its governmental headquarters. At its center lies a majestic stone castle that is home to the royal family, the nobility, and their advisors. The castle is patrolled by the most elite soldiers, and its imposing fortress—complete with towers, battlements, and arrow slits—offers a formidable defense against outsiders. Safeguarding the royal family is essential for the kingdom's survival.

Beyond the castle building, the bustling peasants, market vendors, and roaming castle soldiers provide a constant hum of daily activity. A small network of roads twine around the castle in order to connect the stables, barracks, market storefronts, and all other aspects of city life. Walking along the dusty streets, your ears fill with the sounds of gossiping neighbors, enterprising musicians, and the clack of horse hooves trotting past on the cobblestones as merchants, residents, and soldiers come and go. A perfume of baked bread, fireplace smoke, market spices, and hay saturates the air. This small city is the hub of the entire kingdom.

Encircling this small city is a stone wall that is monitored day and night by castle guards, and an iron gate in this rampart is the only point of entrance to the city and the castle grounds. Residents and visitors must pass through this inner gate in order to leave the city, and then must prove their citizenship again—or their worthiness—in order to re-enter. The inner gate is raised and lowered as necessary throughout the day and is kept closed at night for security.

Outside this inner gate, past the royal family's farms and other small villages, is a second wall. This outer wall is immense and encompasses the entirety of the royal's property. The royal property is the nexus of the medieval kingdom and is home to those with Fire superpowers.

Superpowers of the Fire Realm

Much like an actual fire, the superpowers of the Fire Realm can range from a single flickering flame to a deadly blaze. Flames are not static–rather, they are constantly moving and changing direction. In the medieval kingdom, these superpowers would be used to determine who was worthy to enter the Fire Realm for royal business. In modern life, fire superpowers are used to protect our hearts and enrich our interactions and relationships with people. We all have the superpowers of the Fire Realm, but not all of us have a fire power as our strongest constitutional superpower. Those who do have a fire superpower as their strongest are able to connect and relate to people more easily than those with a constitutional superpower from another realm.

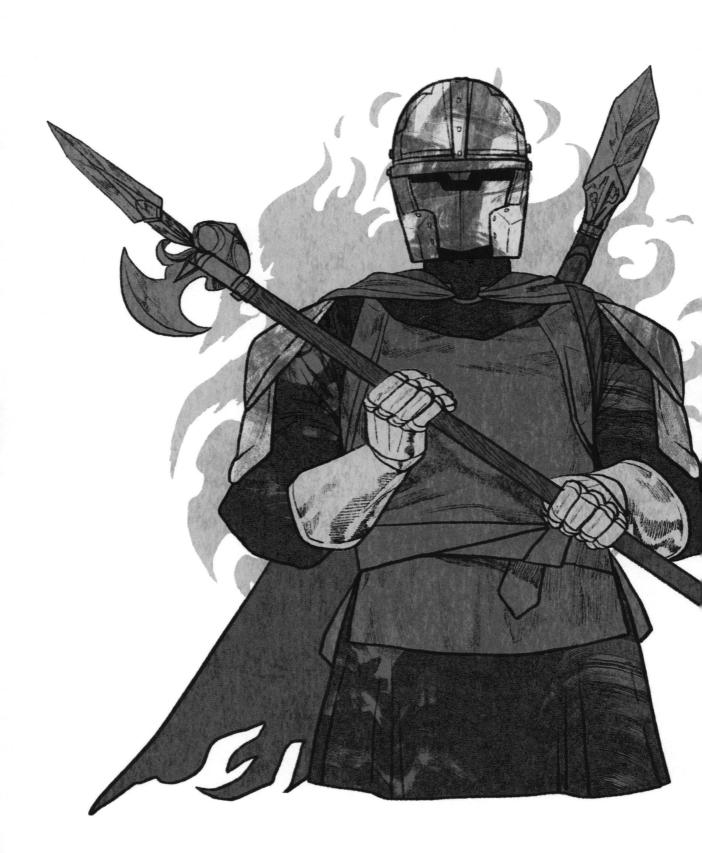

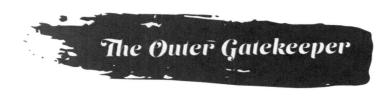

The Outer Gatekeeper

Meditation:

The World is all gates, all opportunities, strings of tension waiting to be struck.

–Ralph Waldo Emerson

Lexicon of Power

Superpower:	The Outer Gatekeeper
Realm:	Fire
Gifts:	Developing a robust social circle; networking
Superpower in Excess:	Exhaustion, inability to develop close relationships
Weakening Realm:	Water
Superpower when Weak:	Inability to network and socialize
Amplifying Realm:	Wood

In the metaphorical medieval kingdom along the outer Fire Realm wall, soldiers are posted as lookouts for approaching visitors. A gate would be housed along this wall near a junction of roads that connect to the other four realms. This gatehouse would have sentries posted for security. Those who want to enter this outer gate could range from artisans hoping to sell their wares, farmers bringing their harvest, families who want to reconnect, or political allies hoping to strengthen relationships. Of course, the sentry would also have to be on the lookout for thieves, spies, and all others seeking trouble. The sentry needs to stay alert in order to decide who can enter the kingdom.

In modern life, our outer energetic gate is constantly being tested. Whenever we interact with those with whom we don't already have established, close relationships, we decide whether to allow their energy past our walls and allow them entrance to our energetic being. For example, if your outer gate is strong and functioning appropriately, you will keep it closed to the angry energy of an impatient driver on your commute. Conversely, if you cross paths with a friendly neighbor who compliments you, your gate should be opened in order to let in the kind energy. Each moment with another being impacts our energetic boundaries. The gift of knowing when to open our energetic gate comes more easily to some than it does to others. Those who have the Outer Gatekeeper superpower as their primary temperament are adept at networking. They are the social butterflies of the world. We all have the capacity to connect with others, but those with this gift are masterful at it. Unfortunately, social media encourages the constant use of this outgoing superpower, and it has become the most fashionable super suit to wear, often to the neglect of the other eleven super suits.

Weakening an Outer Gatekeeper's Superpowers
(Use the gifts of the Water Realm—Courage and Wisdom)

When the Outer Gatekeeper super suit is worn too frequently, it is time to reevaluate those they've allowed past the gate and into their kingdom. Are all those that have been granted access truly worthy of being in the kingdom? There is a safety risk to the kingdom if the Outer Gatekeeper is not screening appropriately for worthy connections. In excess, an Outer Gatekeeper is constantly seeking connection and warmth from others. This can sometimes lead them to overstep social bounds: think fawning hostess, meddling matchmaker, or smarmy salesperson. Water superpowers are the natural kryptonite to Outer Gatekeepers because their powers lie in the appropriate use of wisdom, quiet, and daily effort.

There are many ways to weaken an excessive Outer Gatekeeper and they will vary with every individual. Take time to journal or reflect on the following questions:

What benefits might you experience taking a break from social media for a period?

_____

_____

_____

_____

_____

Meditate on those you've allowed in your social circle. What thoughts come to mind?

_____

_____

_____

_____

_____

When was the last time you had a one-on-one conversation with a friend and were fully present (e.g., you put your phone away and resisted the urge to post about your time together)?

_____

_____

_____

_____

Amplifying an Outer Gatekeeper's Superpowers
(Use the gifts of the Wood Realm—Vision and Direction)

When one needs encouragement to wear the Outer Gatekeeper super suit, they should head to the Wood Realm. Wood energy develops the ability, strength, and purposeful direction to make a plan to connect with positive people that share your interests. Applying wood energy involves channeling frustration into decisive action and creating a vision for the future.

How might this look for you? Take time to journal or reflect on the following questions:

When could you dedicate time to connect with those that might expand your horizons?

_____

_____

_____

_____

Make a list of people you would like to contact or groups and associations you would like to join and haven't yet.

_____

_____

_____

_____

When was the last time you planned a get-together with friends you haven't seen in a while in order to reconnect?

_____

_____

_____

Additional Thoughts

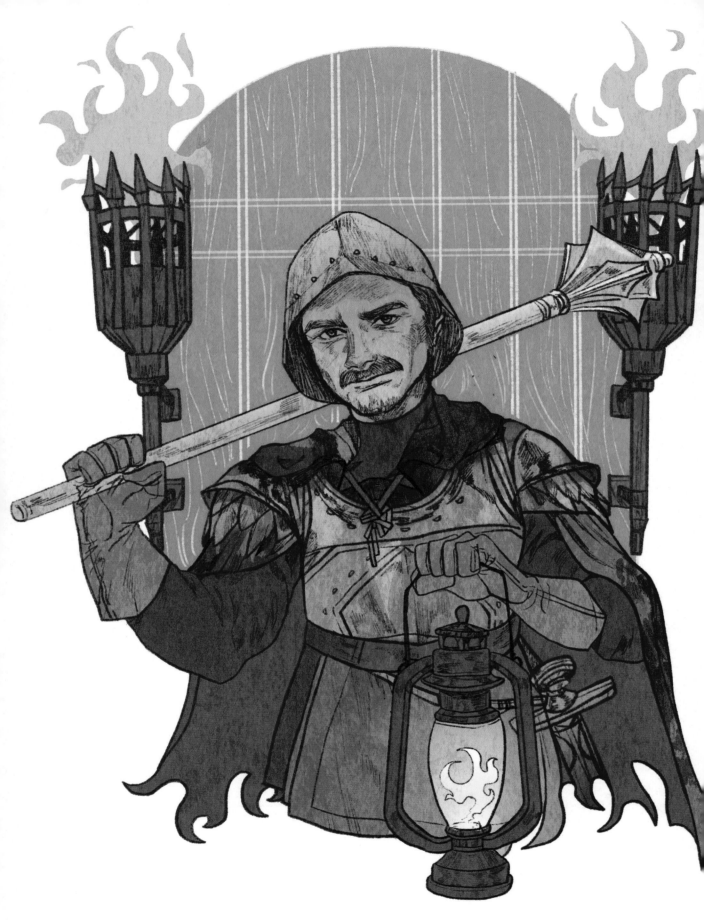

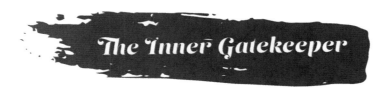

The Inner Gatekeeper

Meditation:

Above all else, guard your heart, for everything you do flows from it.

−Proverbs 4:23

Lexicon of Power

Superpower:	The Inner Gatekeeper
Realm:	Fire
Gifts:	Close circle of friends and family
Superpower in Excess:	No discernment of inner circle
Weakening Realm:	Water
Superpower when Weak:	Loneliness
Amplifying Realm:	Wood

Many may be permitted through the outer gate and cross the Fire Realm's land, but not everyone is allowed entrance to the castle city. It is a privilege to enter the city, because of the proximity to the royal family. To enter the medieval kingdom's castle city, visitors need to pass through the inner gate. The Inner Gatekeeper must filter for those who are worthy of entrance. The inner gate should only be lifted for those who can prove citizenship or royal family business. Many who choose to come to the city would like a meeting with the royal family, but not everyone is permitted an audience. If the Inner Gatekeeper were to lift the gate for everyone, the royal family would not only be completely overwhelmed by the volume of visitors, but there would also be no filter for those who might intend to do harm. On the contrary, if the gate is always kept closed, the Fire Realm city's businesses would suffer, the royal family would miss important kingdom news, and citizens would become isolated from the rest of the kingdom.

As humans, when we decide to allow someone to become close to us—to turn into more than just a casual acquaintance—we're choosing to lift the gate to our inner energetic being. This is an important step in relationship building because we are essentially allowing them to know more about our inner selves. Lifting the inner gate requires vulnerability. In the medieval kingdom, once the gate is lifted, the best opportunity to keep out trouble has passed. In modern life, when we let someone become close to us, we not only have the potential to develop a loving relationship, but we also open ourselves to the possibility of heartache.

Inner Gatekeeper superpowers offer many benefits. The Inner Gatekeeper superpower allows you to see a person not only based on external factors, such as appearance, occupation, or connections, but also to identify the nature of a person's spirit through intuition. This superpower allows all of us to recognize our emotional boundaries and know whether a person is safe and when they should be brought into our inner circle.

Weakening an Inner Gatekeeper's Superpowers
(Use the gifts of the Water Realm—Courage and Wisdom)

If the inner gate is left open, the entire kingdom is jeopardized. A person who lets their guard down and shares too much of themselves without proper discernment, risks allowing people to get close to them that may not have their best interests at heart. If one's Inner Gatekeeper superpower is not screening properly, this is a call to visit the Water Realm. The Water Realm specializes in quiet, and with quiet comes wisdom. Spending quiet time alone provides reflection and the ability to reassess current relationships. This can be a fix to a broken inner gate.

If your Inner Gatekeeper needs kryptonite, take time to journal or reflect on the following questions:

Review times when you have felt hurt or disappointed by someone close to you. Do you still share your story the same way with them?

_____

_____

_____

_____

_____

How much of your life do you share with others? Are you comfortable that they will respect what you have shared with them?

_____

_____

_____

_____

_____

Think about who is your best friend and why.

_____

_____

_____

_____

_____

Amplifying an Inner Gatekeeper's Superpowers

(Use the gifts of the Wood Realm—Vision and Direction)

Alternately, an inner gate can malfunction when it is kept closed inappropriately. Those who do this are the folks who never let anyone close to their inner selves. This may happen for many reasons, but a perpetually closed inner gate also jeopardizes the safety of the kingdom. We all need at least one person in our inner circle. If an inner gate is closed too frequently, it's best to seek the strength and direction of the Wood Realm. Wood superpowers help provide clarity to a misguided or surly Inner Gatekeeper by channeling that frustration in more productive and beneficial ways.

If you wish to apply wood superpowers to amplify an Inner Gatekeeper, take time to journal or reflect on the following questions:

What qualities are important to you in a close relationship?

_____

_____

_____

Is there someone you enjoy spending time with but haven't made an effort to get to know better?

_____

_____

_____

Who are those that you've allowed to know you best? When is the last time you called them?

_____

_____

_____

Additional Thoughts

_____

_____

_____

_____

_____

_____

_____

_____

_____

_____

_____

_____

_____

_____

_____

_____

_____

_____

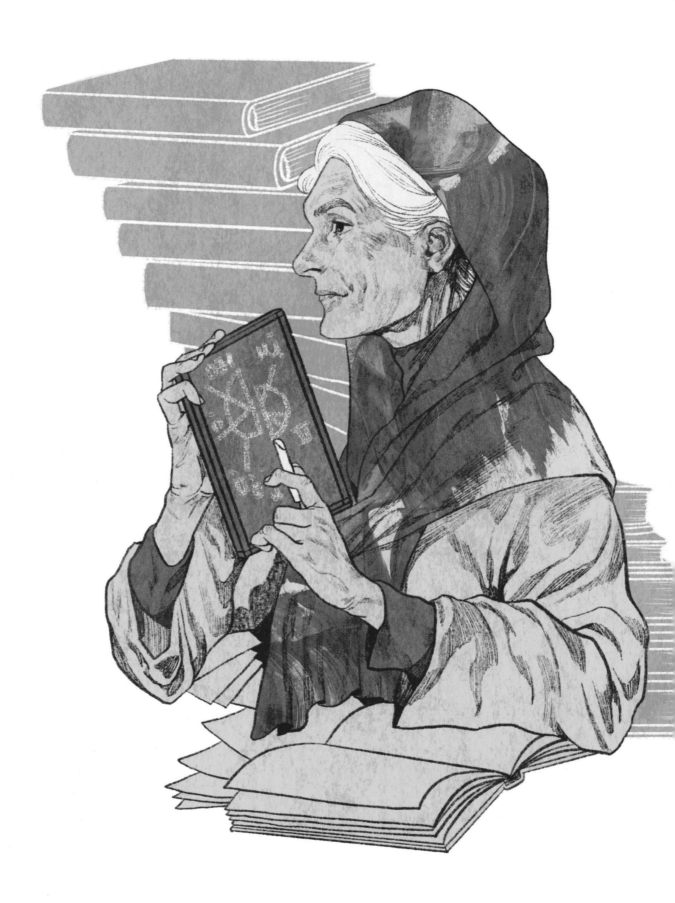

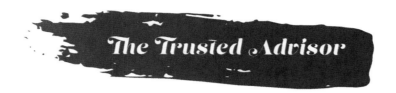
The Trusted Advisor

Meditation:

He who does not trust enough, will not be trusted.

—Lao Tzu

Lexicon of Power

Superpower:	The Trusted Advisor
Realm:	Fire
Gifts:	Sorting life choices appropriately
Superpower in Excess:	Stubborn convictions
Weakening Realm:	Water
Superpower when Weak:	Inability to choose, or regret over life choices
Amplifying Realm:	Wood

Once a visitor with royal business has passed through both the inner and outer gates of the kingdom, they will be brought to meet with the Trusted Advisor. The Trusted Advisor holds an esteemed position because they have a close relationship with the royal family. Advisors listen carefully and sort through each visitor's message in order to get to the heart of the matter.

Not only do Advisors screen visitors' messages for good intentions, but they also advise the royal family on official kingdom policy. One earns the position of a Trusted Advisor by demonstrating an ability to sort through alternatives and possible outcomes in order to find the best solution to a question or problem. Those with this superpower are known for their discernment, propriety, good pattern recognition, and the ability to weed out irrelevant information. Only the most beneficial and purest of messages can be discussed in person with the royal family, and the Advisor has that authority.

The Trusted Advisor is the subconscious mind coaching us during every moment of the day to be our most authentic selves. As humans, we feel best when we are being true and honest. This can be difficult in modern life. There are many internal and external forces at work that can derail us from showing our true person. Social or emotional pressures to dress, act, or be different from one's authentic self can compromise our values. When we feel that we are not being authentic, our personal kingdom suffers.

We all have the capacity to listen to our inner voice and to wear the Trusted Advisor super suit, but there are those who wear it with greater ease and grace than others. These are the folks who know their heart's desire most clearly. This means that they can make difficult life decisions or choose between comparable alternatives without second-guessing themselves. They have little regrets over their life choices because they know in their hearts that the choices they made were authentic to their true selves. This is like a wise guru that sorts through life's options and has the ability to analyze different potential outcomes to make the best decision.

Weakening a Trusted Advisor's Superpowers

(Use the gifts of the Water Realm—Courage and Wisdom)

When a Trusted Advisor suit is overworn, the inner voice may become regimented, and one's convictions may become stubborn. It's important to listen to one's inner voice, but part of the gift of the Trusted Advisor is to check in and recognize that the subconscious message may change over time. The inner voice may now be counseling toward different lifestyle choices, friendship groups, politics, or careers than it previously had. And if we don't tune in to these different messages, we can become stuck in past convictions. When a Trusted Advisor super suit has become stubbornly outdated, it is time for a visit to the Water Realm. Water superpowers can soften or wear down a headstrong, misguided Trusted Advisor by applying life wisdom gleaned through experience or quiet reflection. Applying water energy to weaken a Trusted Advisor requires spending time quietly listening to other people to understand their viewpoint.

How to apply water energy to weaken a stubborn Trusted Advisor will vary with each person. Take time to journal or reflect on the following questions:

Have you noticed a pattern in the types of people that keep showing up in your life? Consider if there is a lesson to be learned from them.

_____

_____

_____

_____

_____

When listening to someone else, are you listening deeply or waiting for your chance to speak?

_____

_____

_____

_____

Ask yourself what challenges your convictions. Are you open to hearing the other side?

_____

_____

_____

_____

_____

Amplifying a Trusted Advisor's Superpowers

(Use the gifts of the Wood Realm—Vision and Direction)

When one has trouble making life choices and forgets to wear their Trusted Advisor super suit, this is a call to visit the Wood Realm. Wood superpowers give direction and offer insight into *how* to go about life. For example, if someone is having difficulty deciding which college to attend, wood energy can be applied by making a list of pros and cons for each choice. Wood superpowers amplify weak Trusted Advisors by offering counsel with regard to planning and decision-making.

As individuals, we will all apply wood energy differently. Take time to journal or reflect on the following questions:

Where could you seek guidance on issues that are important to you?

_____

_____

_____

Meditate on past decisions and actions that have worked well. Why do you think they were successful?

_____

_____

_____

Create a simple list of pros and cons in regard to a major life goal, or make a vision board for a project you're working on.

_____

_____

_____

Additional Thoughts

_____

_____

_____

_____

_____

_____

_____

_____

_____

_____

_____

_____

_____

_____

_____

_____

_____

_____

_____

_____

_____

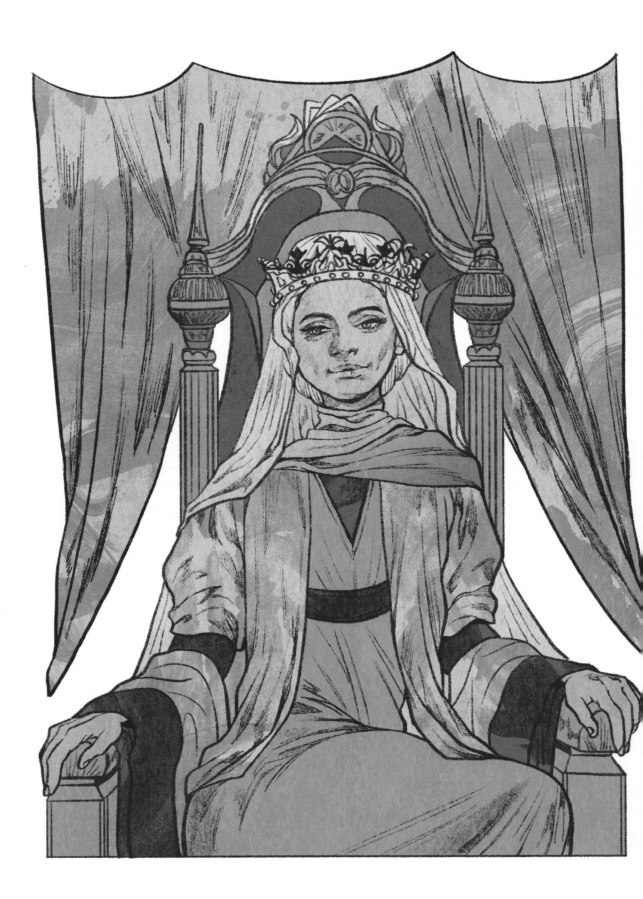

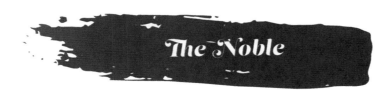

The Noble

Meditation:

Wherever you go, go with all your heart.

–Confucius

Lexicon of Power

Superpower:	The Noble
Realm:	Fire
Gifts:	Authenticity; being true to oneself
Superpower in Excess:	Self-righteous
Weakening Realm:	Water
Superpower when Weak:	Feeling lost, not knowing oneself
Amplifying Realm:	Wood

In the medieval kingdom, the nobles of the royal family have the ultimate power. Their rule ensures the overall safety and success of the kingdom. Citizens of the kingdom look to the nobles of the royal family for law and cultural values. When their edicts and rulings are in the best interests of their subjects, the whole kingdom flourishes and continues on in peace. But if there are uprisings or degradations in royal policy, the whole kingdom will suffer. The Noble's job is to see the kingdom in its true light and to adjust policy or to administer reprimands as necessary.

The Noble of the medieval kingdom is a metaphor for each person's heart. The heart of a person is their true self, and a person's most authentic self can be difficult to discern when faced with pressures to conform to societal and familial prejudices, outward appearances, and other circumstances. Modern life holds many distractions and conflicting messages. When acting in accordance with the missives of one's true self, we are most at peace physically and emotionally.

We all have the Noble superpower within us; however, there are those who wear this super suit more frequently than others. Those who hold a Noble superpower as their greatest strength are recognizable in today's world by their unflinching dedication to their values. Their actions, words, and lives are based on a combination of the messages of their inner voice, intuition, and internal value system. Noble superpowers are used when we must stand up, do the right thing, and look out for others. Nobles stand out because of their vigorous efforts toward the causes that they champion, which ultimately give their life meaning. They feel strongly for others on a deep level. In general, they are the ones you would identify as having a big heart.

Weakening a Noble's Superpowers
(Use the gifts of the Water Realm—Courage and Wisdom)

When a Noble super suit is worn too much, an individual can overextend their energy toward so many causes—or focus so acutely on one—that they lose sight of what they find to be truly important. Feeling deeply for others can upset them on a grand level. Focused on others' pain, they may have difficulty being present in their own lives and blind to the feelings of those close to them. This is like an uncontrolled fire spreading outward in multiple directions. Water superpowers help channel and direct a noble's fierce convictions into manageable goals through contemplation and wisdom.

If you need to apply the wisdom and quiet of water energy as weakening power to a Noble, take time to journal or reflect on the following questions:

How do your everyday actions affect those closest to you?

_____

_____

_____

_____

_____

Meditate on the wisdom that you've gained from helping others. Does the same level of energy still needs to be extended?

_____

_____

_____

_____

_____

Reflect on how you can be fully present with those you love.

_____

_____

_____

_____

_____

Amplifying a Noble's Superpowers

(Use the gifts of the Wood Realm—Vision and Direction)

When a Noble super suit is difficult to wear, wood superpowers can present a broader perspective. Seeing the big picture clarifies the role that a Noble superpower can play in order to champion a cause. Wood energy is all about creating a vision for the future and taking action. Amplify Noble superpowers with wood energy through planning and decision-making.

In order to apply wood energy and amplify a Noble superpower, journal or reflect on the following suggestions:

Visualize what your successful contribution to a cause might be and write down action steps necessary to achieve it.

_____

_____

_____

_____

Make a list in descending order of things that you care most deeply about (your heart's desire).

_____

_____

_____

_____

Develop a daily time management plan to evaluate what areas need more time and focus.

_____

_____

_____

Additional Thoughts

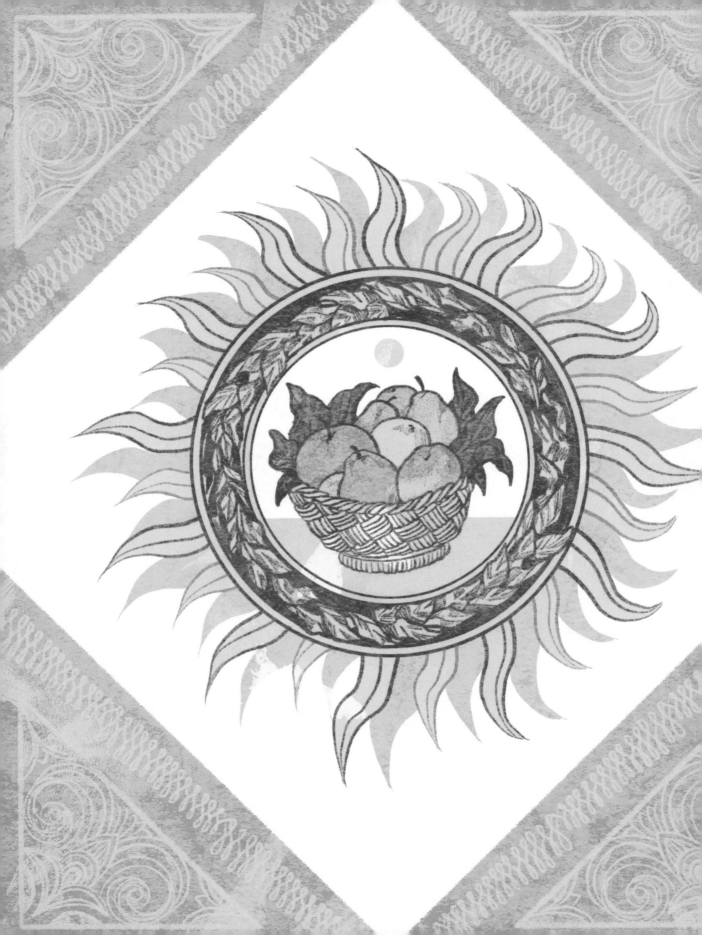

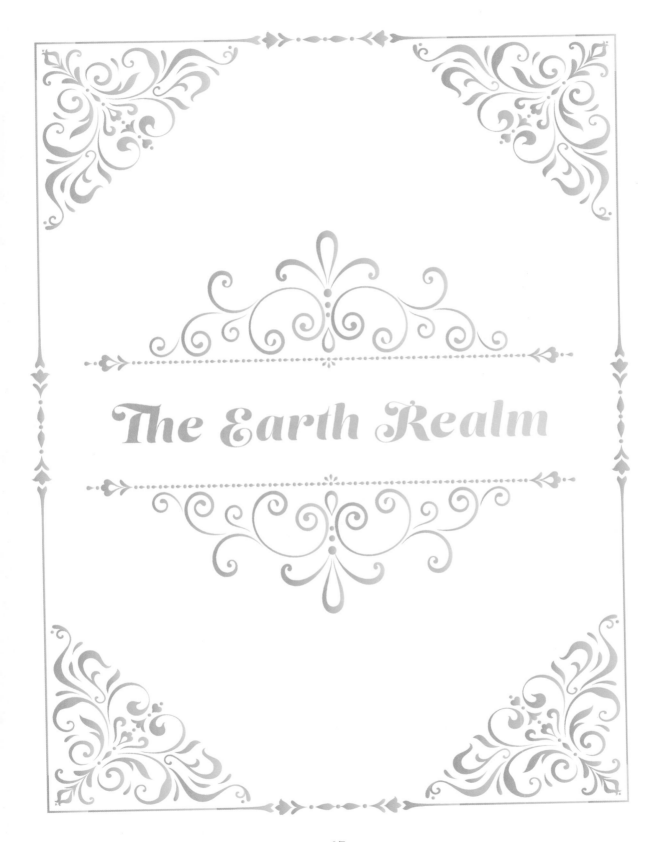

The Earth Realm

Gifts of the Realm
Sympathy – Understanding

As you travel away from the Fire Realm, wide expanses of farmland come into view, framed by groves of apple and pear trees. Beyond the orchard, rows and rows of crops ready for harvest fill the air with the sweet scent of plump berries, vine-ripened tomatoes, and flowering herbs. The gentle breeze carries a melody: the songs of farm laborers, the chirps of crickets, and the cooing of mourning doves. Eventually, thin lines of chimney smoke appear in vertical columns in the air, enticing weary travelers to venture into a large village filled with expansive farmhouses. Travelers are graciously welcomed in the Earth Realm, and hospitality is a key tenet of Earth culture. As the food source and culinary capital of the kingdom, the realm is known for its bountiful harvest feasts.

Superpowers of the Earth Realm

Those with superpowers of the Earth Realm harness a circular, rounded energy that is much like the orbit of the earth around the sun, or a mother rocking their child to sleep. The movement is a smooth back-and-forth from the periphery back to center. With this energy, one can focus on details, people, and events from many different angles. This circular energy calls forth with its power to process food, information, and all of life's experiences. In fact, those with the superpowers of the Earth Realm are the nurturers and thinkers of the kingdom.

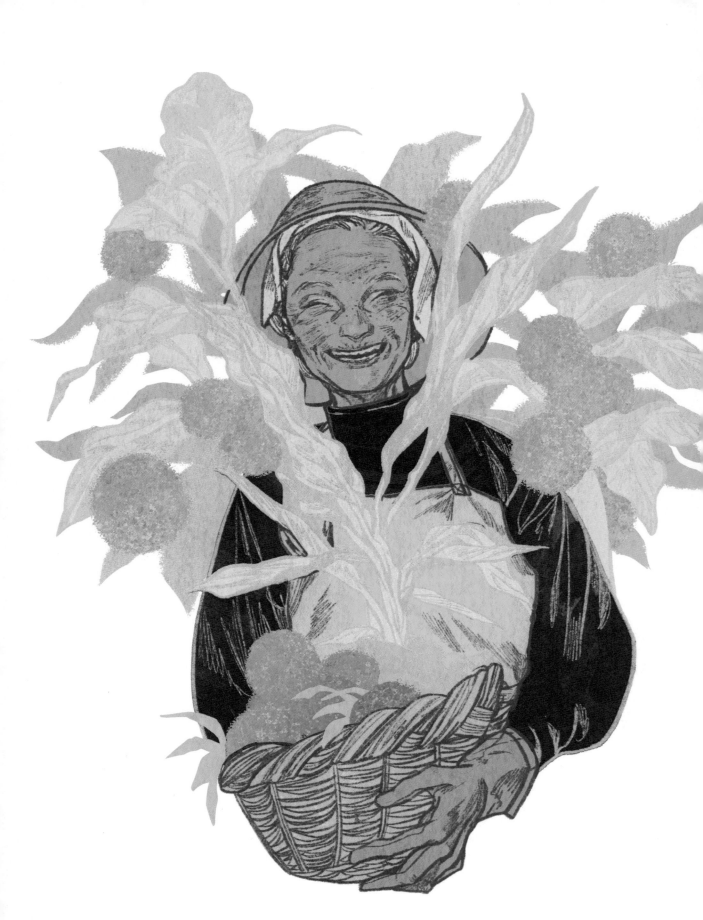

The Gardener

Meditation:

Consideration for others is the basis of a good life, a good society.

—Confucius

Lexicon of Power

Superpower:	The Gardener
Realm:	Earth
Gifts:	Nurturing others
Superpower in Excess:	Worry, smothering
Weakening Realm:	Wood
Superpower when Weak:	Rejecting sympathy
Amplifying Realm:	Fire

Gardeners play a huge role in the success of the kingdom, as they are responsible for feeding its people. And this is not an easy task. Gardeners require patience. Caring for plants—or any living creature, for that matter—demands tenderness and mindful attention. It also calls for a certain level of education over the subject matter. Knowing when to water, prune, or simply move a plant can be specific to each variety. Different creatures require different foods, handling, and housing. Humans all share a similar physiology, and yet we are unique due to our genetics, culture, personality, emotional state, and a myriad of other factors. In order to truly care for another being, one must understand their needs. Every being is needy in some form or another.

Gardeners are like the richest soil of the earth, furnishing the optimal growing environment. They can discern and provide for the needs of others. Often, these people are good listeners. They are the go-to people when you want someone just to listen and not necessarily to offer advice. Through the act of carefully listening, they can understand and therefore envision themselves in the position of the person speaking to them. This requires care and effort. Compassion is a superpower gift that we all have to offer, yet those who have this superpower as their primary constitution will also have it as their greatest strength.

Weakening a Gardener's Superpowers
(Use the gifts of the Wood Realm—Vision and Direction)

When a Gardener superpower's rounded, circular energy becomes excessively out of balance, they may try to over-nurture themselves or others. Everyone likes to feel cared for, but no one likes to feel smothered by attention. Too much invasive caretaking can make the other person question themselves unfairly. Wood energy controls this excess by setting clear boundaries and limitations.

If you need meditative wood energy to weaken excessive Gardener superpowers, take time to journal or reflect on the following prompts:

Reflect on a time where you thought you could take care of yourself but were made to question your ability to do so.

_____

_____

_____

_____

_____

Consider the balance between the time you schedule for yourself each day and the time you spend on others. Does the balance seem appropriate?

_____

_____

_____

_____

_____

To identify over-nurturing, think of the nurturing actions and words you use toward others. Are there any that would frustrate or anger you if they were aimed toward you?

_____

_____

_____

_____

_____

Amplifying a Gardener's Superpowers

(Use the gifts of the Fire Realm—Social Connection, Vulnerability, Discernment, and Love)

With underuse of a Gardener superpower, one may draw attention to their suffering, but then in the same breath reject any offer of sympathy. Those that do not accept help or sympathy from others may think they're being selfless, but instead they may actually be insensitive to those trying to share their pain and connect with them. When one buckles under the weight of bearing their own suffering without help or sympathy from others, it is time to visit the Fire Realm. Fire people love to connect with others and are excellent at lifting burdens through camaraderie and laughter.

If you need to apply fire energy to amplify a Gardener superpower, take time to journal or reflect on the following prompts:

What close friend or family member could you call about your troubles?

_____

_____

_____

_____

Reflect on your feelings about a personal issue that you are dealing with. How could you ask for and accept help without judgment.

_____

_____

_____

_____

Meditate on how it feels to care for other people. When was the last time you had that feeling?

_____

_____

_____

_____

Additional Thoughts

_____

_____

_____

_____

_____

_____

_____

_____

_____

_____

_____

_____

_____

_____

_____

_____

_____

_____

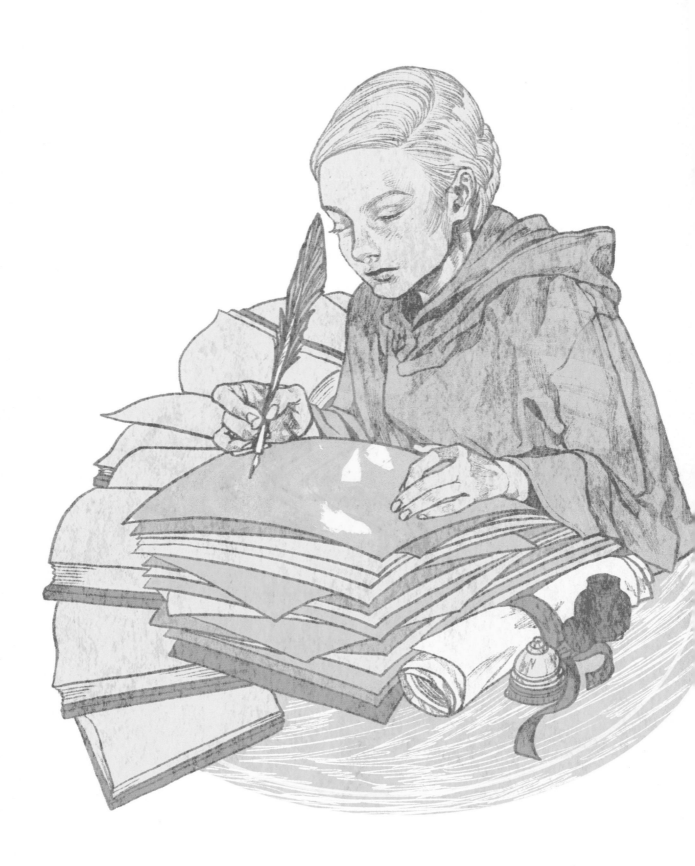

The Scholar

Lexicon of Power

Superpower:	The Scholar
Realm:	Earth
Gifts:	Processing ideas; understanding life
Superpower in Excess:	Anxiety, over-thinking
Weakening Realm:	Wood
Superpower when Weak:	Inability to process life's moments
Amplifying Realm:	Fire

Scholars serve an important and revered role in the ancient kingdom. Based on their extensive education, Scholars could make sense of current events and history, as well as explain both everyday and complex concepts to those who might have been less educated. Their role was to provide help in terms of processing and understanding the events of the time. By doing so, Scholars were able to minimize fears of new and strange events, which provided comfort and ease in the kingdom.

A Scholar is someone with an aptitude for study. Not everyone enjoys learning new things or examining new subjects. However, we are called to do so during practically every moment of our lives. Each new moment brings change in one way or another, and these changes need to be digested and understood as we continue to move forward in life. Some moments are easily processed, like tasting new food, hearing a funny joke, or brushing your teeth. Others are much heavier and take time to digest. Scholars have a natural affinity for examining these moments from many different angles. Given that the Earth Realm's energy is rounded, Scholars will take an issue and examine it from all possible viewpoints. They usually have sound judgment because they consider all sides of an issue before making a decision.

Weakening a Scholar's Superpowers
(Use the gifts of the Wood Realm—Vision and Direction)

Scholars can suffer from excessive worry. Worry is a negative side effect of the Earth Realm; this goes for both Gardeners and Scholars. All of the rounded energy that is used to care for another or consider all sides of an issue can continue in a constant loop of anxiety, if not managed properly. By ruminating about all possible outcomes, Scholars and Gardeners can get stuck in what-if scenarios that prevent them from moving forward. Wood energy is a natural control to this rounded energy as it is linearly directed and forward focused. With its clear vision for the future, it will charge through the stagnant excess of circular energy with a plan for change.

To apply wood energy to weaken excessive Scholar superpowers, take time to journal or reflect on the following prompts:

Visualize and write down the best possible outcome for every worry.

_____

_____

_____

_____

Wood energy is about taking action. Take a long walk in nature or choose another form of exercise.

_____

_____

_____

_____

_____

_____

Make a list of things you need to accomplish and cross them off when done.

_____

_____

_____

_____

_____

_____

Amplifying a Scholar's Superpowers

(Use the gifts of the Fire Realm—Social Connection, Vulnerability, Discernment, and Love)

Excessive thinking and processing of information can cause one to feel disconnected from the world. Not knowing about what's going on in the world, even on a very basic level, can cause loneliness and alienation to set in. This is a call to visit the Fire Realm. Fire superpowers will provide the spark needed to reengage in life. Fire superpower's primary life focus is to engage with others, and by doing so, it can coax out weak Scholar energy and help develop an interest in the world again.

If you need to apply fire energy to amplify weak Scholar superpowers, take time to journal or reflect on the following questions:

What team, class, or other group interests you?

_____

_____

_____

_____

_____

Which friend or family member would lift your spirits if you spoke with them now?

_____

_____

_____

_____

What is a funny podcast or comedy that might make you smile?

_____

_____

_____

_____

_____

Additional Thoughts

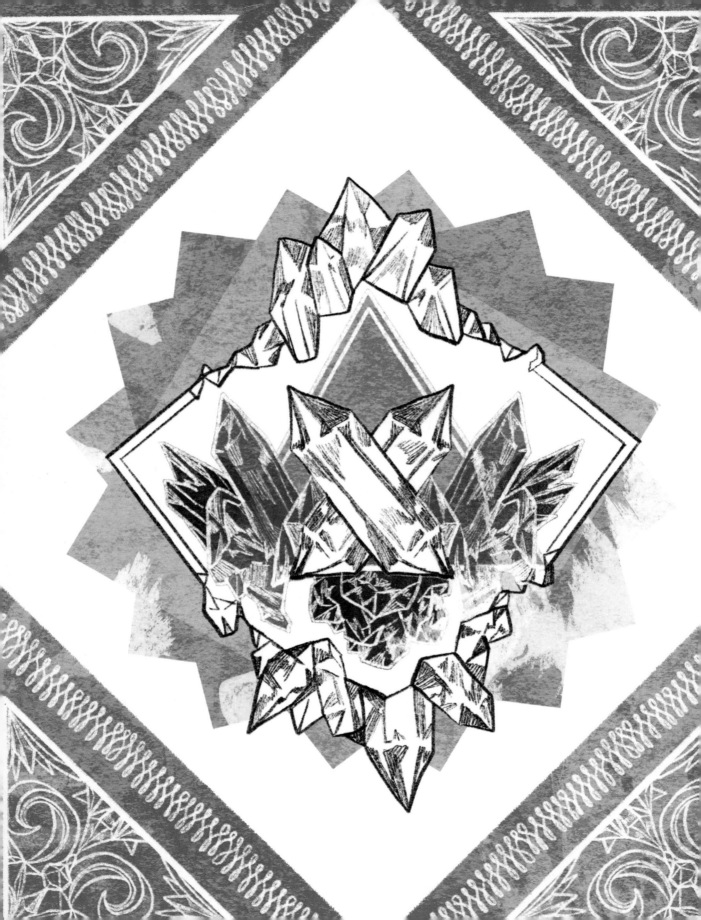

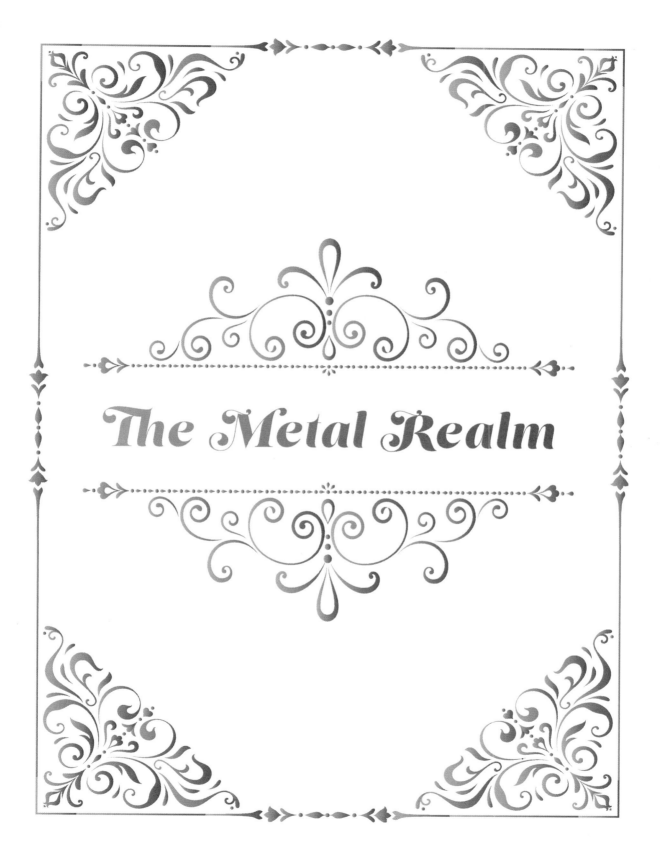

The Metal Realm

Gifts of the Realm
Acknowledgment – Loss

From the Earth Realm, travelers head toward the Metal Realm. Beyond the endless, rolling farm fields, the path becomes sprinkled with rocky gravel. Mountains appear on the horizon–dark, looming, and purple one moment, and glistening white the next, as the sun catches the quartz crystals in the rock face. The lush farmland of the Earth Realm is a distant memory as the natural landscape becomes dotted with large boulders and only a few stark trees.

The Metal Realm is the treasury of the kingdom, as their mines produce the most precious of metals. It's a difficult process to acquire the precious metals of the kingdom, and because of this, the residents of the Metal Realm have developed a strong appreciation for what is truly important in life. A chief cultural principle of the Metal Realm is to treasure what is valuable and avoid wasting excess time or energy.

Superpowers of the Metal Realm

Those from the Metal Realm are the inspirers and judges of our world, as both inspiration and judgment require cutting to the heart of the matter. Inspiration comes from the spark of creativity or from finding the value in the mundane. Judgment has the power to let go of something that does not serve you well. This energy is like the vulture that can soar higher than any other bird and yet nourish itself on earth by picking through what others would consider waste.

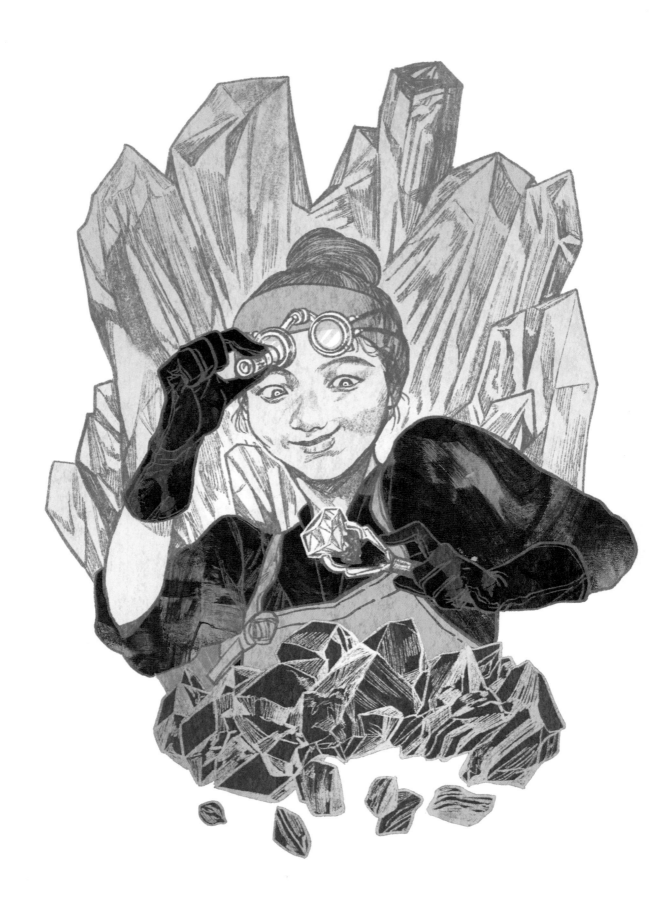

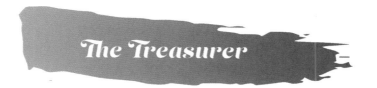

The Treasurer

Meditation:

Everything has beauty but not everyone sees it.

−Confucius

Lexicon of Power

Superpower:	The Treasurer
Realm:	Metal
Gifts:	Inspiration; knowing what is of value in life
Superpower in Excess:	Hoarding tendencies
Weakening Realm:	Fire
Superpower when Weak:	Losing sight of what is truly valuable in life
Amplifying Realm:	Earth

In our medieval kingdom, Treasurers assign value to the precious gems and metals gathered from the mine. They have the unique ability to determine the worth of each stone. It's a gift to be able to discern what is of value, especially when it involves finding the gem in the middle of a rough stone. The Treasurer's job is to ensure the richness and wealth of the kingdom by making sure that the items kept in the vault are only the rarest, most exquisite, and most valuable. By doing so, they maximize the fortune of the kingdom. This is done not by inundating the vault with tons of stones, but rather by using their acumen to add the greatest financial impact by including only the most treasured pieces.

Those who have the Treasurer as their constitutional superpower find the spark of creative genius, pearl of wisdom, witty insight, or unseen beauty in what others may consider to be mundane. They take everyday items, thoughts, and concepts, and then create beauty out of them. We all have this ability, but there are those of us who call this power to themselves with simple and routine ease. This is the aha moment of inspiration that comes upon us when a new person, exciting idea, or clever joke enters or emerges from our personal kingdom. Like finding a bright pink shell on an otherwise sandy brown beach, the directional energetic movement of this superpower mimics the quick inhalation of a sudden discovery.

When a Treasurer's superpower is balanced and healthy, they have a tidy living space with personal items that create a sense of contentment. Out of balance, a Treasurer will begin to retain items that might resemble what they value but are not exactly in line with what they truly merit. Over time, these subtle shifts in standards of worthiness lead to an over-accumulation of items. This can ultimately bring on hoarding tendencies, as their perception of what is important becomes increasingly skewed. What were once clear lines distinguishing beauty and usefulness translate to crammed closets, overstuffed drawers, and chaotic workspaces.

This hoarding tendency can also apply to relationships and thoughts. When a Treasurer's super-power is at its strongest, the people in their lives are like the bright shiny jewels in the kingdom's vault. Each person brings beauty, kindness, creativity, joy, or some sort of comfort to the Treasurer. However, with the overuse of this super suit, judgment may become skewed. Those friendships or relationships that were once uplifting could become stale, wearing, or depressing. It may take the form of holding a grudge against someone they feel has wronged them, obsessing over a familiar memory or outdated idea, or clinging to anything that is negative or harmful to them in some manner. It could also manifest as reliving a triumph or success that has long since passed. Again, these shifts can be subtle transitions over time, so the transformation from cultivating an enriching crowd to accumulating an unconstructive one can occur easily and without mindful realization.

Weakening a Treasurer's Superpowers

(Use the gifts of the Fire Realm—Social Connection, Vulnerability, Discernment, and Love)

Treasurers, at their strongest, value each present moment and do not surrender their powers to the past. If the Treasurer super suit has become outdated or overworn, it is time to visit the Fire Realm. Fire superpowers can melt away stubborn tendencies by offering new conversation, camaraderie, friendship, or simply the trust needed to let go of things that no longer serve them. Fire superpowers inherently find joy and live fully in each moment. By spending time with others, a new script of discussion, experiences, and places can shift one away from the stagnation of living in the past. It offers an opportunity to rewrite or move on from outdated or overplayed memories or physical objects.

There are many ways to weaken an excessive Treasurer with fire energy. Take time to journal or reflect on the following prompts:

Is there something new you have been wanting to try (gym class, hobby, book club, etc.)?

_____

_____

_____

_____

_____

Meditate on the selfless feeling you had when you last spent time with someone you love.

_____

_____

_____

_____

_____

To bring out inner inspiration, consider if there is a new creative endeavor you could try (e.g., drawing, sculpting, writing a story, or playing an instrument).

_____

_____

_____

_____

_____

Amplifying a Treasurer's Superpowers

(Use the gifts of the Earth Realm—Sympathy and Understanding)

Metal energy is about honoring what currently has value or once had value in your life. Experiences, thoughts, and relationships need to be digested and understood in order for a person to learn from them and move forward. Loss is an inevitable part of life. The Earth Realm's rounded energy provides perspective to consider and appreciate moments from all sides before releasing them to memory. Earth's soil houses metals, and like a mother that provides a safe and secure play area, earth energy allows a space for acknowledgment of what was once important to you.

Every individual will apply earth energy a little differently to amplify a Treasurer superpower. Take time to journal or reflect on the following prompts:

Reminisce over past experiences or relationships and consider what you learned from them or what gifts you received.

_____

_____

_____

_____

_____

Consider what new things you've learned, special moments you've had in your day, or things that you are grateful for.

_____

_____

_____

_____

_____

Take or collect pictures of special places, items, or people that are meaningful to you.

Additional Thoughts

_____

_____

_____

_____

_____

_____

_____

_____

_____

_____

_____

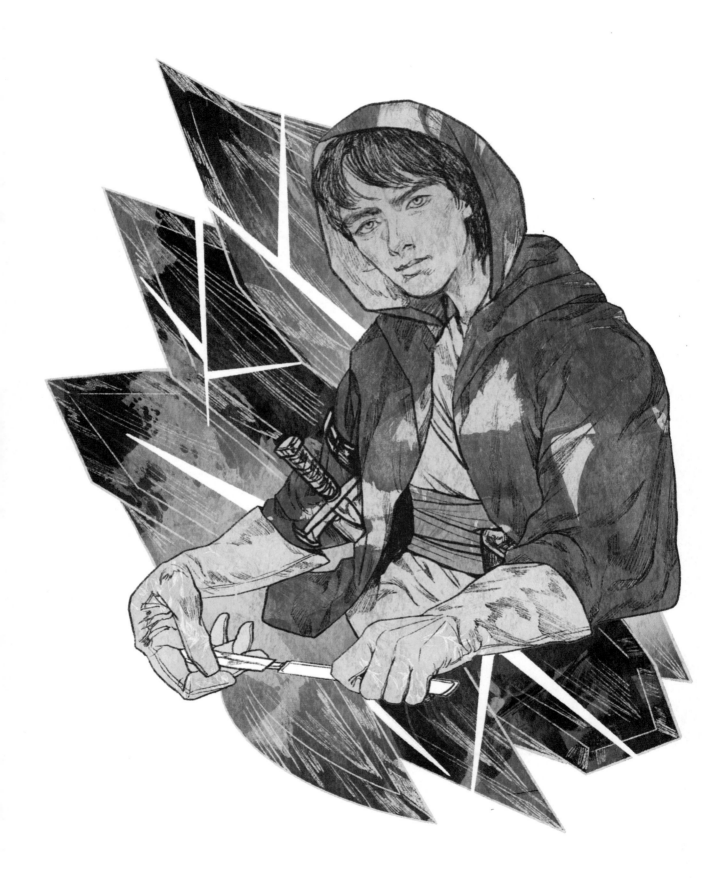

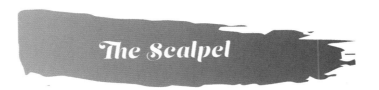
Meditation:

Simplicity is the ultimate sophistication.

—Leonardo da Vinci

Lexicon of Power

Superpower:	The Scalpel
Realm:	Metal
Gifts:	Judgment; ability to leave or discard what does not serve
Superpower in Excess:	Cutting people or things out of life inappropriately
Weakening Realm:	Fire
Superpower when Weak:	Not embracing self-worth
Amplifying Realm:	Earth

Miners in the Metal Realm use sharp metal tools to carve a tunnel network through underground rock. Using their instruments, they remove huge amounts of debris with incredible skill and speed. But their job is a difficult one, because they need to be able to quickly identify whether the rocks they are discarding might hold precious gems or minerals. Most of the materials they encounter are waste. These workers are valued because they stay focused even after hours of chipping away. Where others might become complacent, bored, or lazy, these workers are able to recognize a gem even after hours of discarding rubble.

In today's world, those with a Scalpel superpower know exactly what to cherish as valuable in their life and will cut out without a second thought what is too costly for them to keep. This is a powerful gift. Due to technological advances and easy access to material items, historic notions of value are being rewritten every moment. This pertains to everything from modern translations of family units, friendship groups, styles, ideas, political thoughts, and so on. The world is ever-changing. Those with a Scalpel superpower navigate this modern world and find what resonates as beauty in both form and idea with more satisfaction than others.

The Scalpel superpower is used in life to judge what is of value. Those wielding this power do so like a sharp knife honed to perfection. They will discard old photos, once-treasured clothing, or even heirloom family china if it does not speak to them as necessary in their present life. This judgment also applies to those they keep in their circle. They can walk away from an acquaintance, friendship, or lover more easily than others when they have determined these individuals no longer serve their best interests. In general, those who hold a Scalpel superpower cut people, ideas, or things out of their lives with less difficulty than those with a different temperament.

Others may perceive those who wield the Scalpel superpower as being snobby or stuck-up, but this is not actually the case. They are not intentionally looking to disregard people; they simply will not notice others if they're not on their radar of value. Unlike a fire superpower, who is constantly seeking human camaraderie, Scalpel superpowers are not interested in others for the sake of companionship. If they are to invest in a relationship, there must be a greater meaning to the affiliation.

Weakening a Scalpel's Superpowers

(Use the gifts of the Fire Realm—Social Connection, Vulnerability, Discernment, and Love)

When a Scalpel super suit is worn too often, an excess of judgment will arise. Sharper verdicts and more hurtful criticisms can erupt in place of balanced incisiveness, apparent when they lash out with biting commentary. This excessive judgment may also be turned inward toward oneself, translating over time into feelings of unworthiness or harmful thoughts. Fire superpowers soften the sharp metal of a Scalpel superpower. Laughter and small moments of joy can help erode the stagnation of excess judgment. Those with Fire superpowers will naturally gravitate toward anything joyful.

Here are simple examples of how to apply fire energy as kryptonite to Scalpel superpowers. Take time to journal or reflect on the following prompts:

What is something you find inherently joyful (e.g., watch a funny video, play with puppies or kittens, laugh with a friend, sing or dance)?

_____

_____

_____

_____

_____

Think about those less fortunate than you. How could you help them?

_____

_____

_____

_____

Ask a friend for their opinion and consider it with an open mind.

_____

_____

_____

_____

Amplifying a Scalpel's Superpowers

(Use the gifts of the Earth Realm—Sympathy and Understanding)

If a Scalpel super suit is rarely worn, it's time to visit the Earth Realm. Earth superpowers can help sharpen and strengthen a Scalpel. Scalpels need the courage and conviction to cut, without remorse, the things from their life that do not serve them well. Earth energy is rounded; therefore, using earth energy requires examining an issue from all possible viewpoints in order to arrive at a better understanding. It's easier to make a decision when you've considered all sides of an issue. By taking the time to objectively assess an object, relationship, or thought, clearer judgment will surface. The Earth Realm provides this nurturing thought-processing to boost the confidence of a weak Scalpel superpower.

Applying the amplifying power of earth energy to a Scalpel superpower will be different for every individual. Take time to journal or reflect on the following questions:

What do you find to be comforting?

_____

_____

_____

_____

_____

Who in your circle understands you best? Why?

_____

_____

_____

_____

_____

Which good friend could you ask for a "confidence boost" over coffee and know that you can believe what is said?

_____

_____

_____

_____

_____

Additional Thoughts

_____

_____

_____

_____

_____

_____

_____

_____

_____

_____

_____

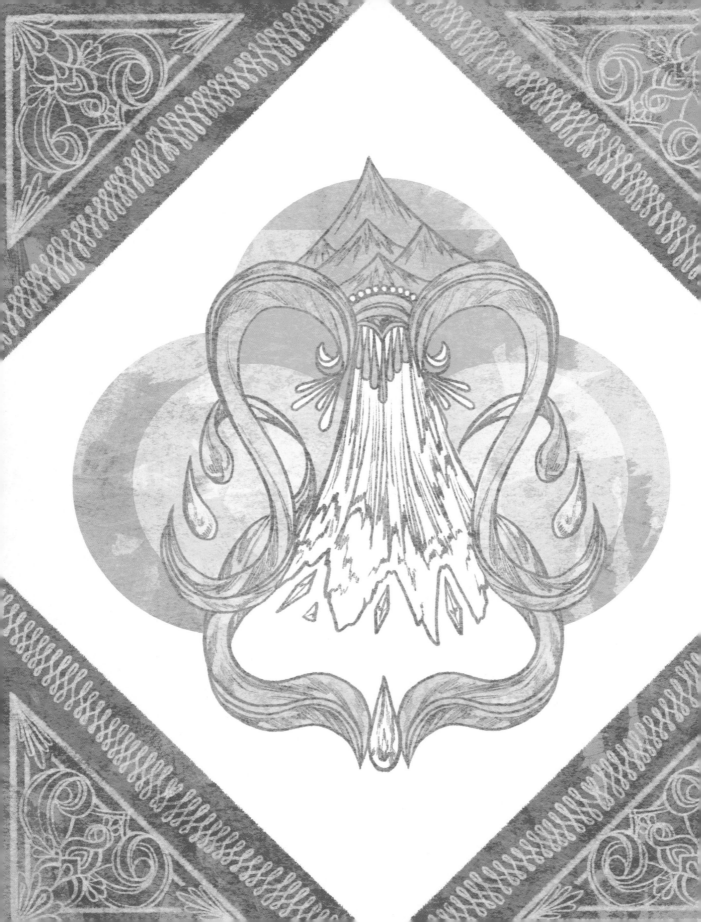

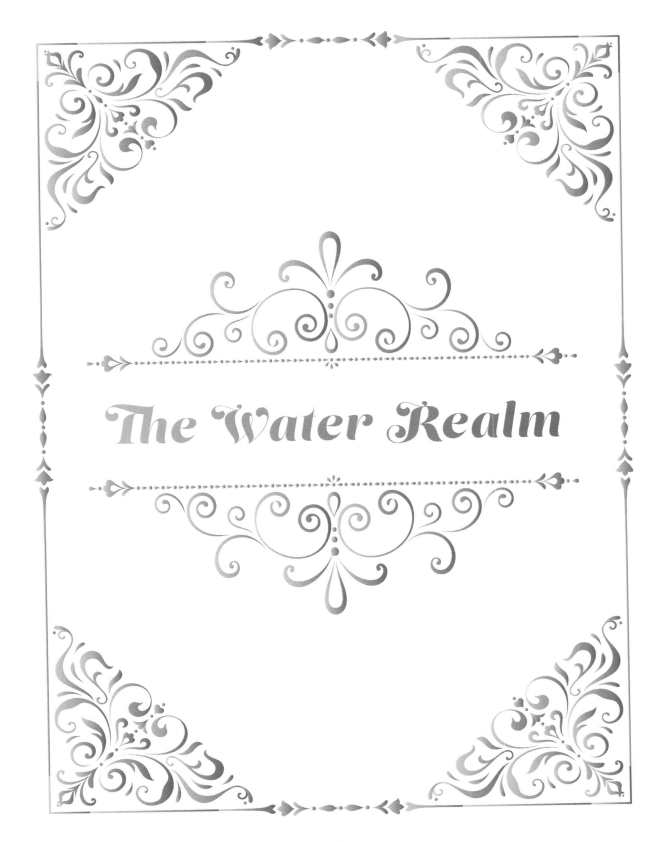

The Water Realm

Gifts of the Realm
Courage – Wisdom

The path away from the Metal Realm leads over the mountain peak and down the other side to the Water Realm. As the windward side of the mountain, the Water Realm has much more precipitation, both rain and snow. After you cross over the snow-covered mountaintop, an evergreen forest appears, and the sound of rushing water fills the air. Years of spring runoff from the heavy snowfall have carved a deep river trench that eventually falls hundreds of feet to sea level. This stunning waterfall can be a trickle in winter or a roaring, thunderous crash in early spring. The waterfall lands into a deep pool at the base of the mountain.

From the top of the mountain, the village buildings of the Water Realm look like tiny ants circling the plunging pool of the waterfall. The pool is expansive and covers a huge area at the foot of the mountain. Those who live in the Water Realm either work toward storing and preserving the clean drinking water from the pool or utilizing the force of the waterfall via water mills for the kingdom's power.

Superpowers of the Water Realm

The waterfall and deep pool are the perfect analogies for the two superpowers of the Water Realm: the Torrent and the Vessel. The directional energy of the Water Realm is a descent downward to the ground. As with a waterfall, gravity forces water to seek its lowest level, and unless contained in some fashion, it will not stop. This is like human willpower. Every human has willpower, of course, but those who wear a Water Realm super suit have stronger and more regular drive, self-discipline, and stamina than those who do not. Both superpowers of the Water Realm use the directional force of water energy, but in two distinct ways: knowing when to use its mighty strength and knowing when to preserve its purity. Torrents manage the huge water-driven saw and the grain mills. Vessels focus solely on preserving and storing the pure, clean water of the realm. And both are necessary for the health of the kingdom.

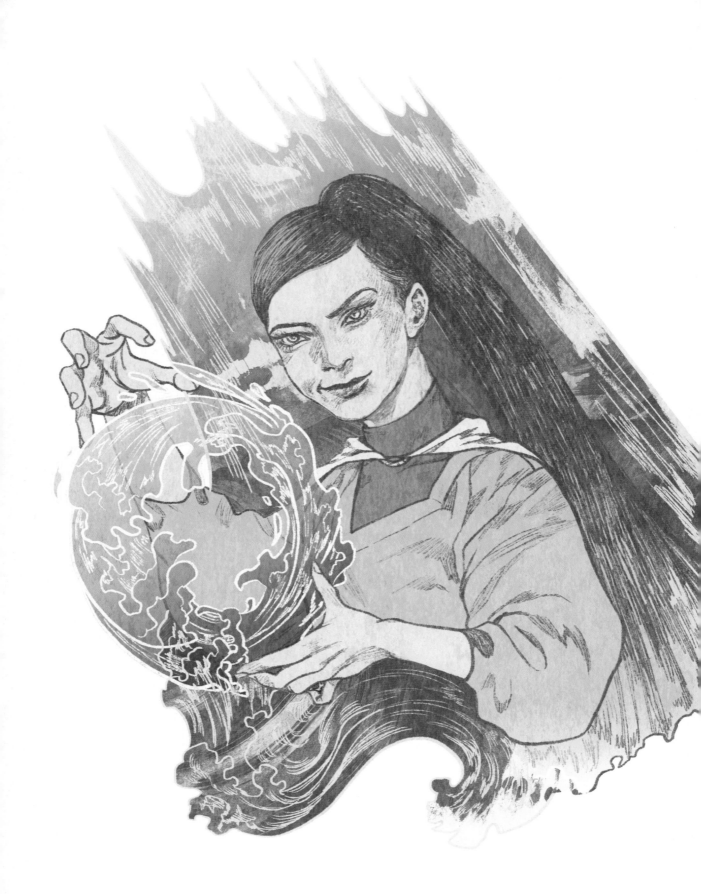

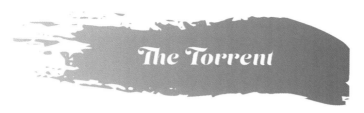

The Torrent

Meditation:

Those who flow as life flows know they need no other force.

−Lao Tzu

Lexicon of Power

Superpower:	The Torrent
Realm:	Water
Gifts:	Willpower and courage
Superpower in Excess:	Fearless, taking inappropriate chances
Weakening Realm:	Earth
Superpower when Weak:	Inappropriately fearful
Amplifying Realm:	Metal

The tall waterfall of the Water Realm generates huge amounts of force. This force is redirected to water wheels at high speeds through a network system of tanks, pipes, and channels. Torrent superpowers work in this industry by making sure that all of the mechanics of the system are working properly and that water energy is conducted as necessary. They quite literally empower the kingdom. It is through their gifts that they can apply the strength of the water toward its most effective use.

Those who wear the Torrent super suit as their primary constitution are driven to perform, and they will push themselves harder than others to achieve their individual goals. Like a huge tidal wave that plows past its normal limits, they will keep going long after others have moved on or given up. Torrent energy is also used specifically toward one's purpose in life. We all have a role to play, and the Fire Realm gives us the edict for our authentic self, but the Water Realm offers the power to bring our purpose into fruition. When we are flowing with our life purpose, life is easier. Time passes quickly, but we enjoy each moment more fully or are simply more present in each moment.

Weakening a Torrent's Superpowers

(Use the gifts of the Earth Realm—Sympathy and Understanding)

Using Torrent energy requires a mix of fear, faith, and courage. This can lead to taking reckless chances or pushing past the limits of one's constitutional energy. The addiction of living in a life-or-death decision frame of mind draws upon reserves of Torrent energy that will eventually deplete the energetic pool. For example, making routine decisions to stay up late, run marathons, or overwork oneself are all activities that are hard to sustain over time. Earth energy offers the ability to process life events before moving on to the next one, as well as the nurturing space in which to consider why an action should be taken. Earth energy is used to provide boundaries and the processing time one needs to choose an appropriate use of life-altering thoughts and actions. Earth energy embodies the spirit of nurturing. When caring for others, you tend to slow time down, earning the space to catch your breath.

To apply earth energy as daily kryptonite to a Torrent superpower, journal or reflect on the prompts on the following page:

How can you best care for yourself today (e.g., make comfort food, take a bath, go to bed early, get up early, call a friend, postpone a non-urgent task, get a haircut, book a massage, read a book, do yoga, etc.)?

_____

_____

_____

_____

_____

How can you care for someone you love today? What simple gifts could you offer to nurture them (e.g., listen deeply, prepare a meal, run an errand for them)?

_____

_____

_____

_____

_____

Who is the best person to listen to you—someone who will understand how you are feeling?

_____

_____

_____

_____

_____

Amplifying a Torrent's Superpowers

(Use the gifts of the Metal Realm—Acknowledgment and Loss)

The other side of courage is fear. When one doesn't wear the Torrent suit, they miss out on opportunities for greatness. Metal energy allows you to see the value in using and fostering courage.

To amplify a Torrent superpower with metal energy, journal or reflect on the following prompts:

Recall a time when you were acknowledged for doing something well. How did you feel in those moments?

_____

_____

_____

_____

Who do you respect most in your life and why?

_____

_____

_____

_____

What gifts have you received through your relationships with others?

_____

_____

_____

_____

Additional Thoughts

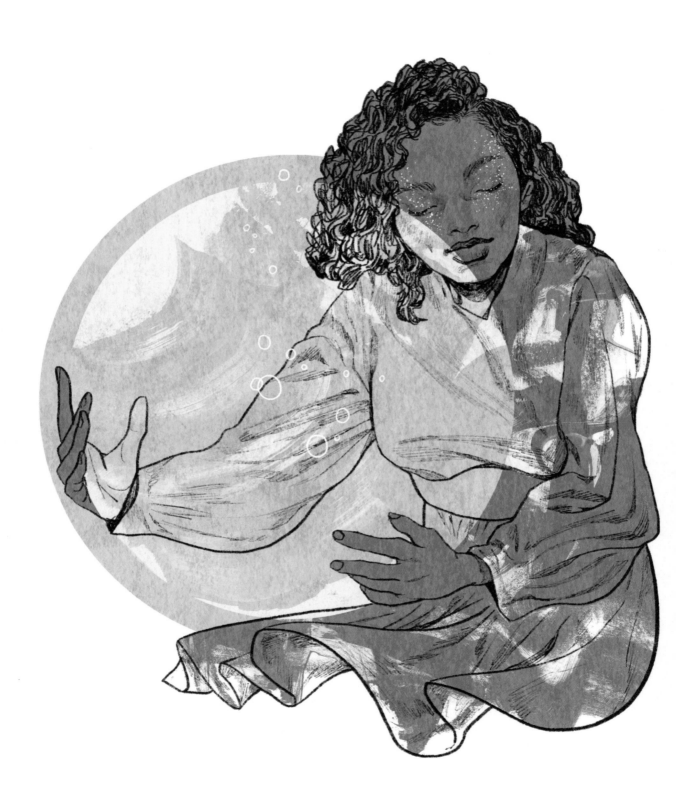

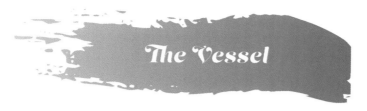

The Vessel

Meditation:

Silence is a source of great strength.

−Lao Tzu

Lexicon of Power

Superpower:	The Vessel
Realm:	Water
Gifts:	Life wisdom
Superpower in Excess:	Misguided faith
Weakening Realm:	Earth
Superpower when Weak:	Inaction
Amplifying Realm:	Metal

Carved over centuries by the pounding of the force of the waterfall, the pool at the base of the mountain appears bottomless. Its depth is unfathomable, and it can withstand even the most torrential season, expanding and contracting with the varying levels of rainfall. The clear water that fills the basin is stored for those who live in the kingdom. Those who collect and preserve this resource, the Vessels, hold an esteemed position in the kingdom. Water from the Water Realm is treasured for its purity and strengthening powers. Vessels know when and how much of this precious reservoir inventory should be stored.

Vessel energy, like that of a Torrent, is the power used to bring one's life purpose to fruition, the accumulated knowledge or life wisdom learned through one's experience or the experiences of others. This Vessel energetic suit is worn when one needs to determine whether further energy is needed in a particular moment. Note that this is different from making daily or instinct-driven decisions. This is either the choice, or need, to draw upon one's life essence in order to move toward one's life goals.

Weakening a Vessel's Superpowers

(Use the gifts of the Earth Realm—Sympathy and Understanding)

Vessels are in charge of holding the reserves of the kingdom. Resisting change and holding on to reserves of energy out of fear can cause the vessel to overflow like a flashflood. Earth energy is used to help contain this excess by considering all sides of an issue and using that understanding to set boundaries and priorities. Look to earth energy when an opportunity to move forward on a life path arises but fear freezes you in place. Not moving forward with your life destiny is destructive in the same way that too much careless action can deplete you. For example, if you are afraid to leave your home, you may never meet your life partner. Earth energy is used in this instance to help us understand why using energy reserves can make a positive life change.

Everyone will amplify a Vessel superpower with earth energy differently. Take time to journal or reflect on the following prompts:

Reflect on a time when you felt steady, centered, and composed in the midst of change.

_____

_____

_____

_____

Take time to learn and understand more about aspects of a situation that make you uncomfortable.

_____

_____

_____

_____

_____

Find a meditation geared toward centering. Practice this meditation to gather your thoughts and senses.

_____

_____

_____

_____

_____

Amplifying a Vessel's Superpowers

(Use the gifts of the Metal Realm—Acknowledgment and Loss)

The Vessel superpower retains some of the fuel used to help bring your life purpose into action. When this reserve is not monitored or spent appropriately, it may become contaminated or be depleted in careless ways. Metals enrich the quality of water by contributing minerals that aid the body's process; however, too much or too little of these minerals could also be harmful. When a Vessel superpower does not monitor the purity of the pool, there's less ability to refresh the kingdom with its gifts. This can translate to a tarnished outlook on life or a loss of purpose. Metal energy reminds a weak Vessel superpower that, similar to a unique gem, a Vessel's role offers immeasurable value and is an integral part of the kingdom.

How this metal energy will be applied will vary with everyone. Take time to journal or reflect on the following prompts:

Think about what unproductive or unnecessary part of your life could be eliminated or cut out to make space for something better.

_____

_____

_____

_____

_____

Acknowledge a time when you performed well. How did that feel?

_____

_____

_____

_____

_____

What areas of your life do you cherish?

_____

_____

_____

_____

_____

Additional Thoughts

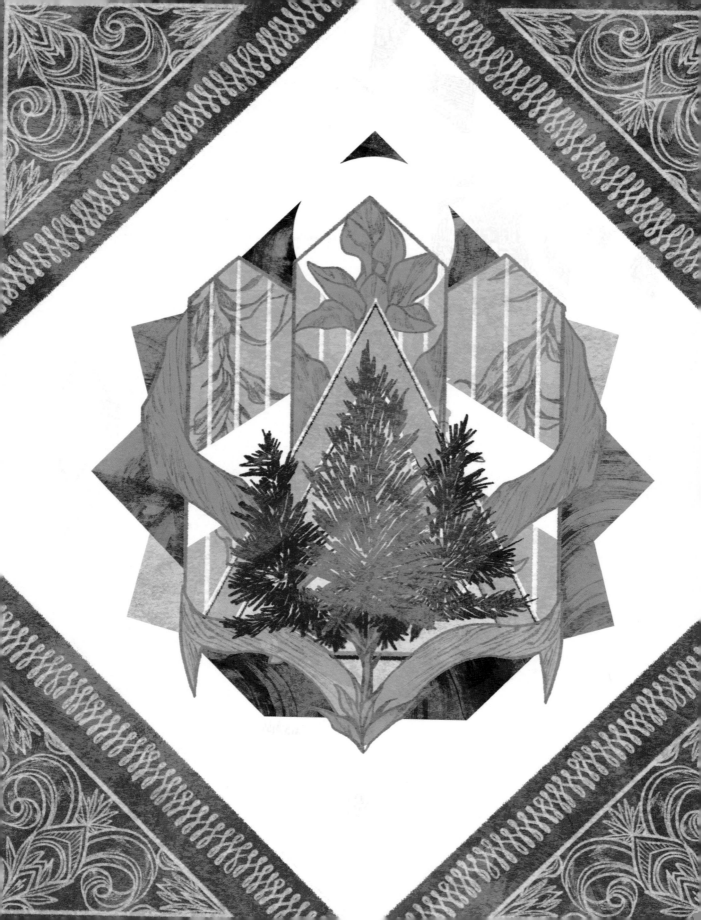

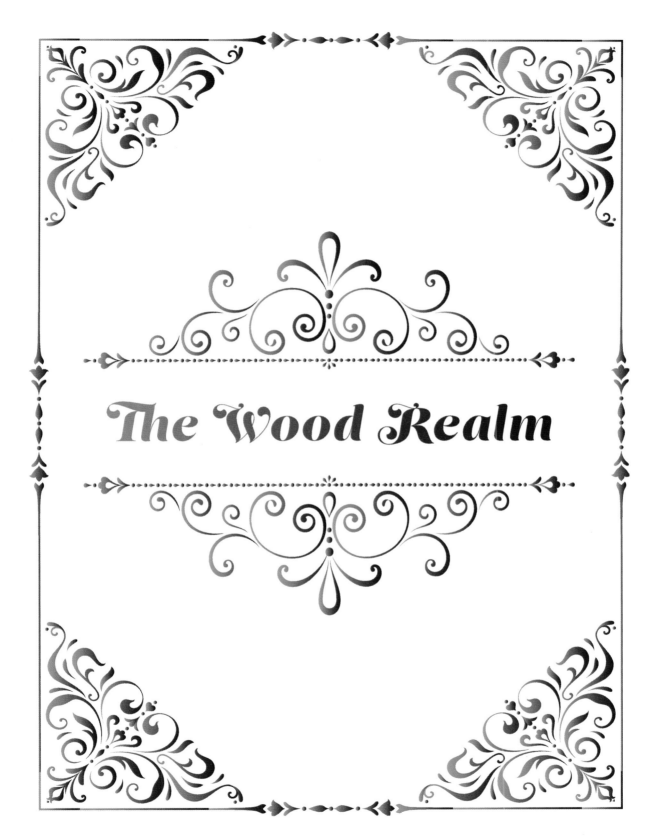

The Wood Realm

Gifts of the Realm
Vision – Direction

In the medieval kingdom, the Wood Realm lies to the east of the Fire Realm and is a verdant forest filled with ancient, colossal trees. The woodland villages are connected by a maze of paths winding through the forest. Superpowers from the Wood Realm harness the power of springtime energy. Living so long within this forest, its residents are gifted with the energetic virtue of wood. They utilize the same force that pushes a tiny seedling up through the ground to meet the sun, an upward-moving energy that calls them forward along their path.

Superpowers of the Wood Realm

This upward-moving energy of the Wood Realm manifests in various ways, but this energy collects and resides in the eyes, culminating in a clear vision for the future. Those with wood superpowers are masterful at planning. Much like a hawk perched high in a treetop, they are able to survey the landscape around them in order to determine the best path forward.

In the modern day, those who resonate with this energy as their strongest superpower feel most comfortable when they have a plan and know the specific steps needed to execute the plan's mission. These are the natural leaders of the world, and they crave structure. These are the people who love to set schedules and keep to them. They like to know what to expect and when things will happen. And, if possible, they prefer to manage every decision involved with the plan.

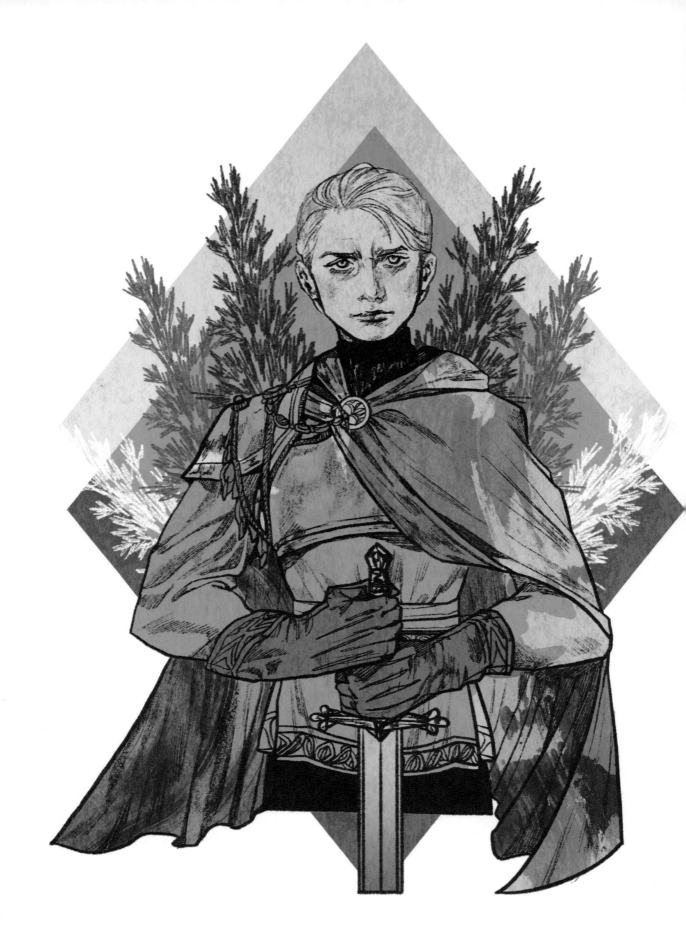

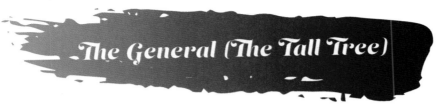

The General (The Tall Tree)

Meditation:

To see things in the seed, that is genius.

–Lao Tzu

Lexicon of Power

Superpower:	The General
Realm:	Wood
Gifts:	Visualizing plans
Superpower in Excess:	Frustration, anger
Weakening Realm:	Metal
Superpower when Weak:	Lack of purpose
Amplifying Realm:	Water

In the ancient kingdom, Generals were the most gifted with strategy. They commanded respect due to their success in terms of mobilizing troops, leading campaigns, and deceiving one's enemy. The success of a General depends upon seeing the big picture of the battle.

The General's superpower is used to visualize plans beyond the everyday. They are like the tall trees of the forest that have the strength and energy to rise high above the ground. Only from this high perspective can a General see all that is happening around them. For example, they can picture the innovative marketing plan, the winning football play, the layout of the building, or the interior design of a room with more imagination and greater success than the average person because they can literally see it in their minds prior to its actual formation. It is a gift of vision and initiative. Like all of the superpowers, everyone has the General at their disposal. Some, however, choose to use the General superpower more often than the other eleven. When a General's superpower is used in its purest force, plans and actions can come together brilliantly and with great ease.

Weakening a General's Superpowers

(Use the gifts of the Metal Realm—Acknowledgment and Loss)

Generals can become bullies with the overuse of their power. As a result, their followers may either abandon them or follow them only out of fear. Generals welcome combative exchanges; they enjoy when others match their aggressive energy. In excess, they will easily demolish anyone who doesn't match them blow for blow. We all have the capacity to lose our temper and become excessive Generals. Metal energy cuts out what is not valuable, such as the excessive anger and frustration that can arise when this suit is overworn. Metal energy reduces the presence of these traits by reminding a General of what issues are truly important. This can deflate and minimize the occurrence of destructive behaviors by focusing on the reason. For example, anger over a loss or failure can be transformed, allowing a General to acknowledge what they could have done better or what lessons they've learned.

Everyone will apply metal to weaken an excessive General superpower differently. Take time to journal or reflect on the prompts on the following page:

When was the last time you asked others' opinions on matters important to you?

_____

_____

_____

_____

_____

Consider what angers or frustrates you most often and ask yourself why.

_____

_____

_____

_____

_____

Properly channeled frustration creates positive change. What frustrates you and how can it be changed?

_____

_____

_____

_____

_____

Amplifying a General's Superpowers

(Use the gifts of the Water Realm—Courage and Wisdom)

If one chooses not to wear the General energetic super suit, they may feel lost and without purpose. The General super suit provides vision, as it provides the "how" with which to go about life. If you want to make a change, take steps (even baby steps) to move toward the achievement of your goal. Water energy supplies the stillness and space you need to contemplate the life wisdom you've acquired. Armed with wisdom, courage will surface and help you to move past your fear of change.

To amplify a General's superpower, journal or reflect on the following prompts:

Recall a moment of bravery that led to a success.

_____

_____

_____

What essential lessons have you learned from leaders in your life?

_____

_____

_____

Visualize having boundless reserves (including time and money). Make a list of positive things you could accomplish in your life, given these resources.

_____

_____

_____

_____

Additional Thoughts

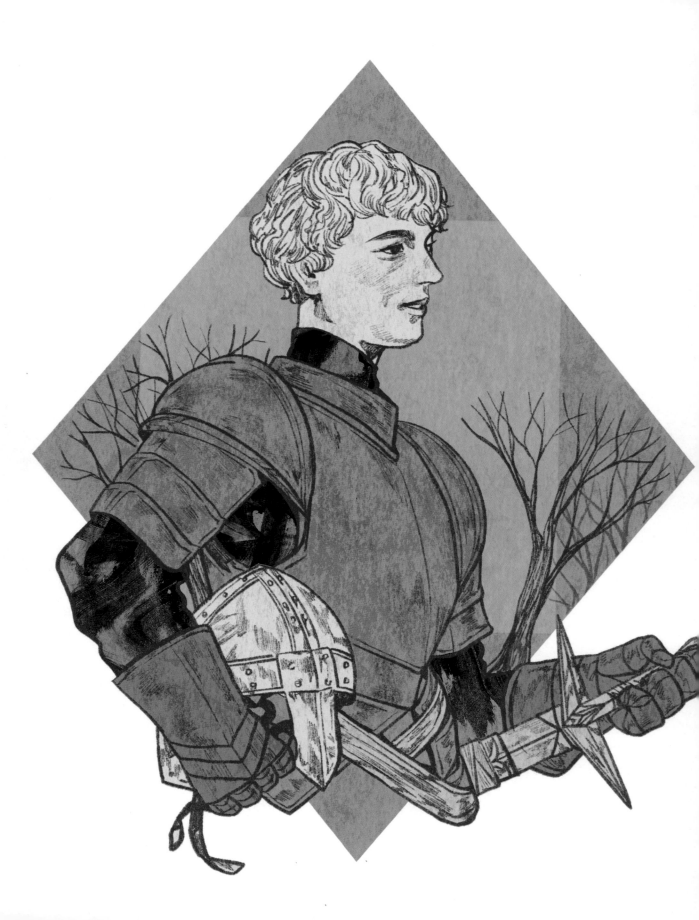

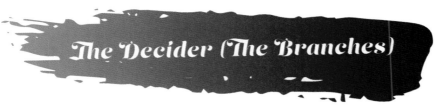

The Decider (The Branches)

Meditation:

Great acts are made up of small deeds.

—Lao Tzu

Lexicon of Power

Superpower:	The Decider
Realm:	Wood
Gifts:	Bringing plans to fruition through decision-making
Superpower in Excess:	Frustration, micro-management
Weakening Realm:	Metal
Superpower when Weak:	Inability to make decisions
Amplifying Realm:	Water

In the ancient kingdom, the Deciders are the officers who implement the battle plan. The General has the long-range vision or an overarching sketch of the plan, but the Decider is the one who actually fills in all of the details. If the General is the tall tree, the Decider is the branch that fills the space in the forest and reaches out from the trunk. An ancient, tall tree will have countless limbs, branches, and twigs extending from its trunk; these branches are like the myriad intricate details of a plan. Big plans take a lot of decisions in order to come to fruition.

In modern life, people make hundreds of decisions each day. What to wear. What to have for breakfast. Which road to take. When to set appointments. And so on. However, unlike those who don't have this dominant superpower, the Decider can do all of this with incredible ease, speed, and accuracy. These are the detail-oriented folks who know how to get stuff done. Whether it's setting up a church schedule to provide meals for needy families, following up with subcontractors on a construction project, or making reservations for a family reunion, Deciders can make plans happen.

Weakening a Decider's Superpowers

(Use the gifts of the Metal Realm—Acknowledgment and Loss)

With the overuse of this superpower, the Decider becomes bossy and controlling and may begin offering opinions or making decisions without being asked. Their frustration at a perceived lack of structure may drive them to overstep social bounds. When the Decider's superpower becomes excessive, they need to experience the tranquil space of the Metal Realm. The Metal Realm culture is based solely on what is most valuable in each moment. Wasting one's energy, or any resource, violates the spirit of the Metal Realm. Metal energy encourages the Decider to breathe, take a moment to relax, and think carefully before wasting energy on action.

Using the gifts of Metal to weaken an excessive Decider's superpowers will look different for every individual. Take time to journal or reflect on the following prompts:

Is there a situation causing unease in your life but it's not yours to handle? Can you let it go?

_____

_____

_____

_____

_____

Who could step in your place as an understudy or backup? Why would you choose them?

_____

_____

_____

_____

_____

Meditate on whether each of your administrative tasks is truly necessary. Is there a way to consolidate or eliminate any busywork?

_____

_____

_____

_____

_____

Amplifying a Decider's Superpowers

(Use the gifts of the Water Realm—Courage and Wisdom)

With underuse of the Decider superpower, decisions become postponed or avoided. The lack of clarity over a decision translates into inaction. The Water Realm provides a space for quiet, rest, and contemplation, which can build reserves of courage you need to face the fear of deciding. Time to rest and recharge can help center a scattered Decider superpower and help them focus.

Everyone will apply the gifts of water energy in their own unique fashion to amplify a weak Decider superpower. Take time to journal or reflect on the prompts on the following page:

Listen to a daily meditation. Record your thoughts afterward.

_____

_____

_____

_____

_____

_____

How can you be fully present while listening to others speak (e.g., put away your phone, turn off the TV)?

_____

_____

_____

_____

_____

_____

When can you make time to simply be still (e.g., sit in a park and watch nature)?

_____

_____

_____

_____

_____

_____

Additional Thoughts

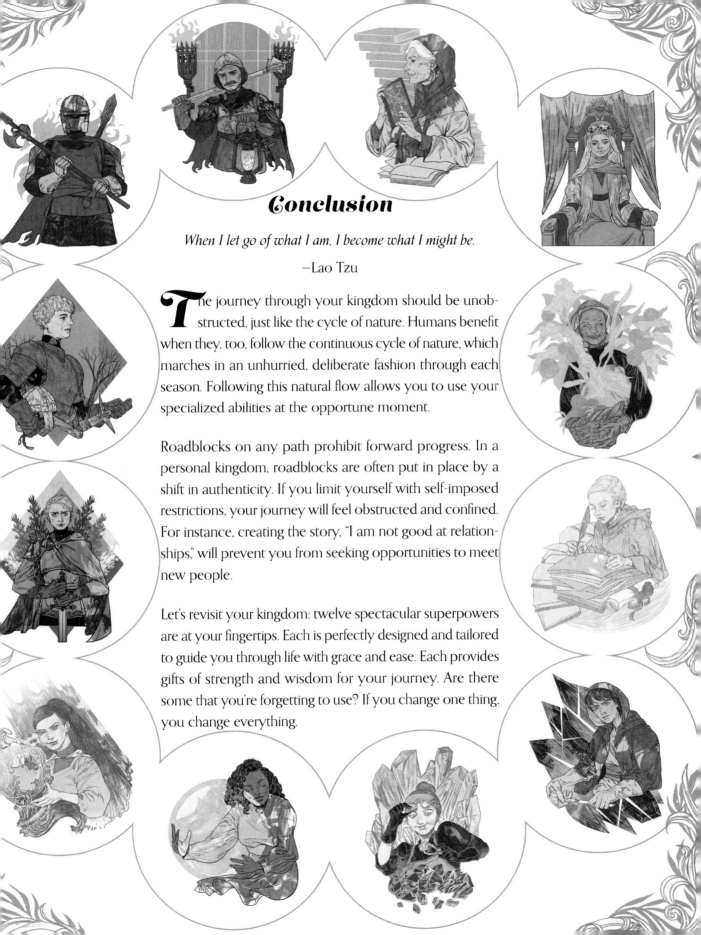

Conclusion

When I let go of what I am, I become what I might be.

—Lao Tzu

The journey through your kingdom should be unobstructed, just like the cycle of nature. Humans benefit when they, too, follow the continuous cycle of nature, which marches in an unhurried, deliberate fashion through each season. Following this natural flow allows you to use your specialized abilities at the opportune moment.

Roadblocks on any path prohibit forward progress. In a personal kingdom, roadblocks are often put in place by a shift in authenticity. If you limit yourself with self-imposed restrictions, your journey will feel obstructed and confined. For instance, creating the story, "I am not good at relationships," will prevent you from seeking opportunities to meet new people.

Let's revisit your kingdom: twelve spectacular superpowers are at your fingertips. Each is perfectly designed and tailored to guide you through life with grace and ease. Each provides gifts of strength and wisdom for your journey. Are there some that you're forgetting to use? If you change one thing, you change everything.

Thanks for Reading

Thank you so much for reading this book. I hope you enjoyed it and found value in the information and perspectives I've shared. Honest reviews are valuable for me as an author, and they help put this book in the hands of other readers. It would mean the world to me if you would take a moment and share your honest thoughts as a review wherever you found this book.

Thanks again,

Mary Krygiel

About the Author

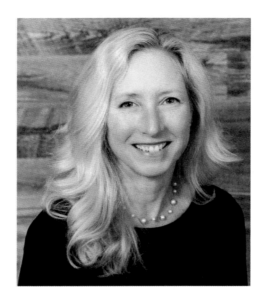

Mary earned a master's degree in acupuncture from the Maryland University of Integrative Health in 2011. As a board-certified, licensed acupuncturist, classically trained in the Law of Five Elements, she has treated many patients in clinical, hospital, and community settings. In each circumstance, she observed that the patient's outward presentation and manner of being contributed to their symptoms. Viewing patients through the lens of her traditional Chinese education, she saw how nature impacts each person's constitution in the way they presented themselves. Interactions can range from effortless to difficult based on a person's use of their twelve energies, as defined by the Law of Five Elements.

Most importantly, however, as a mother to two young adults, she witnessed firsthand the increasing pressure to conform to an overly friendly and excessively engaging presentation on social media. This self-presentation is inauthentic and minimizes our true powers, causing insecurity and self-doubt over time.

Mary came to realize that people's actions, tone, and manner correspond directly with the ancient Chinese understanding of the twelve meridians of energy. These twelve superpowers of humanity, when understood and used effectively, can create greater ease and less stress in each moment of our lives.

Made in the USA
Coppell, TX
10 September 2021

62130657R00069